Oxford Medical Publications

Teaching medical students in primary and secondary care

Anna Wilson.

Teaching medical students in primary and secondary care: a resource book

Dr Sarah Hartley
General Practitioner and Chargé d'enseignement en médecine générale
UFR de Médecine Broussais-Hôtel-Dieu
Université Paris 6
Paris

Dr Deborah Gill
Senior Lecturer in Medical Education
Royal Free and University College Medical School
London

Dr Frances Carter
Honorary Clinical Senior Lecturer
Division of Primary Care and Population Health Sciences
Faculty of Medicine
Imperial College of Science, Technology and Medicine
London

Dr Kate Walters
MRC Fellow
Department of Psychiatry & Behavioural Sciences
Royal Free and University College Medical School
London

Dr Pauline Bryant
Clinical Teaching Fellow
Dept Primary Care and Population Sciences
Royal Free and University College Medical School
London

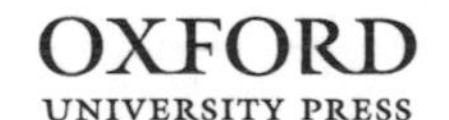

OXFORD
UNIVERSITY PRESS

Great Clarendon Street, Oxford OX2 6DP

Oxford University Press is a department of the University of Oxford.
It furthers the University's objective of excellence in research, scholarship,
and education by publishing worldwide in

Oxford New York

Auckland Bangkok Buenos Aires Cape Town Chennai
Dar es Salaam Delhi Hong Kong Istanbul Karachi Kolkata
Kuala Lumpur Madrid Melbourne Mexico City Mumbai Nairobi
São Paulo Shanghai Taipei Tokyo Toronto

Oxford is a registered trade mark of Oxford University Press
in the UK and in certain other countries

Published in the United States
by Oxford University Press Inc., New York

First published 2003

Reprinted 2004

A catalogue record for this title is available from the British Library

ISBN 0-19-851072-1 (Hbk)

10 9 8 7 6 5 4 3 2

Typeset by Integra Software Services Pvt. Ltd, Pondicherry, India
www.integra-india.com
Printed in Great Britain
on acid-free paper by Antony Rowe Limited, Chippenham, Wiltshire

Foreword

Jane Dacre

Medical Education has changed significantly over the past decade. It has become a much more important area and medical schools are now developing a high level of expertise. External agencies have been developed to ensure that our teaching professionalism flourishes and that our students receive the best education that we can provide. In short it has become accepted that the old clinical adage "See one, do one, teach one" is no longer enough.

The education that students receive in medical school sets the scene for the rest of their medical careers and so should not be taken lightly. This resource book takes the teacher through the stages to becoming a competent professional. It is extremely accessible and refreshingly jargon free. It should appeal to jobbing clinicians as well as those with a specific interest in medical education. It includes clearly written explanations and provides an evidence based journey through medical education.

The book is structured so that it can be used as a resouce but also as a good read and is a mine of useful practical information that should encourage confidence and flexibility in clinical teachers.

It is well referenced for those who want to look into teaching a little further. The book employs an interactive style, which encourages people to learn in an active way—and to pass this skill on to their students.

This is a book that will support our medical and clinical teachers in their teaching of students in primary and secondary care and through this will enhance the experience gained in medical school.

Medical Education will continue to change to reflect changes in medicine itself and advances in educational theory. Those who read this book will be starting from a very strong position to embrace these changes.

We would like to thank our longsuffering families for their support,
and each other for mutual encouragement, coffee and toast.

Contents

CHAPTER 1
Introduction

What is in this book

We will all be asked to teach at some time in our professional lives. If asked to imagine teaching in the medical setting, most of us would think of a large lecture or bedside clinical teaching. However, in the last two decades both medicine and teaching have moved on. Higher patient turnover and the introduction of day surgery have reduced the numbers of patients available for students to clerk in hospitals and increased the amount of teaching done in the community. The change in doctors' hours has affected the firm system, and made it harder for students to feel part of a team. Teachers who can help students come to terms with a more fragmented learning experience are in demand.

Medical teaching has developed to deal with the changes in medical school experience. More doctors have the chance to do regular teaching, and an array of new teaching and assessment techniques are now used in undergraduate and postgraduate settings. You might be asked to facilitate a problem-based learning group, lead a pharmacology seminar, take a group to the skills laboratory, or use videos for consultation skills teaching.

Teaching a course you are familiar with can be worrying, but teaching an unfamiliar course may lead to sleepless nights. Whether you are experienced or a new teacher, this book has been designed to help. Chapters 1–4 have been designed for the new teacher and lead you through the knowledge and skills you will need to teach. Chapter 5 looks at the content of what you teach in greater depth, explaining how to maximize learning using different techniques. Chapter 6 looks at designing effective audio-visual aids, while Chapter 7 looks at how you can modify your teaching depending on the number of students in your group. Chapter 8 deals with the setting of teaching and the challenges of delivering teaching while you continue your clinical work.

More experienced teachers may be asked to design a course, and Chapter 9 offers an introduction. Assessing students is an important part of teaching, and another area where there have been significant changes in the last few years. Chapter 10 covers different types of assessment, helping you to understand how and why they are used, how to assess students accurately, and how to write questions. While we assess students to see how well they have learned, we also need to look at our own teaching and courses as a whole to see whether they are adequate. Without reflection on our teaching, none of us can progress as teachers. Chapter 11 covers evaluation—both using reflection to evaluate our own teaching and looking at simple techniques for evaluating the courses we teach.

Learning in the professions has to be lifelong. This reflects the fact that medicine is continually changing, and that a professional has a duty to remain knowledgeable and competent. Chapter 12 covers some of the issues of continuing professional development, looking at the ways in which professionals learn, at approaches such as mentoring and peer assisted learning, and at appraisal. Teachers need to keep learning too, and the chapter also covers methods of keeping up-to-date, with advice about teaching portfolios, professional associations, useful courses, and how to apply successfully for membership of the Institute of Teaching and Learning.

Because teaching is a discipline in its own right, it has developed its own vocabulary. Many non-teachers find educational jargon confusing. We have tried to avoid unnecessary jargon, and where possible have included explanations in the text. However, there is also a glossary of common educational terms at the end of the book.

How to use this book

You can use this book in two ways: it can be used as a practical guide, and also as a reference book about teaching. It has been designed to be quick and easy to use—it covers all current teaching methods, the common settings for teaching, and helps you deal with different sized groups. Thus if you are lecturing to a large group then look up the section on lecturing and that on large group techniques. If you are teaching clinical skills in the skills laboratory, look up skills teaching and skills laboratories.

If you have not taught before it is worth spending some time going over the contents of Chapters 1–3. Try and plan your first few sessions using the techniques described—and remember that the preparation needed for the first few sessions will take time. With experience you will become much quicker.

Knowing how to do something is only half the story—knowing why can transform your skills. There is a wide educational literature supporting many of the newer teaching methodologies, and experienced teachers often want to know more. We have included further information about the theories behind teaching, and guidance for further reading. You do not need to read these sections when you start to teach, but may want to return to them at a later date and reflect on them in the light of your new experience of teaching.

You will find that we have used icons to signal the different parts of the book.

This indicates a practical tip that will help you in your teaching.

This signals the theoretical sections—reading them will increase your understanding of medical education, but you don't have to read them to be able to teach—you can save them for later.

Teaching medical students well is highly rewarding. Teaching offers variety in clinical routine, and the satisfaction of seeing your students learn, pass their assessments, and eventually become competent clinicians, is hard to beat.

Educational literature is confusing, as it is theory-rich, and evidence-poor (Prideaux and Spencer, 2000). Like all disciplines it has its own jargon, and it is common for educationalists to refer to theories using the names of their authors, rather like clinicians talking about eponymous syndromes.

> I thought of Berger's but wondered about Henoch-Schönlein purpura
> — PRHO

> I think Bloom is too complicated and so I tend to stick to Gagné
> — educationalist

Because many educationalists come from a humanities background, they tend to quote profusely and eclectically in their texts. Scientists may find this heavy going, and conclude that the absence of hard data invalidates the work. Of the six main theories currently in vogue (adult learning, cognitive theory, reflective practice, transformative learning, self-directed learning, and experiential learning) (Kaufman *et al.*, 2000) many are hypothetical, although others (particularly cognitive theory) have convincing support from experimental psychology. As hypotheses, however, they can provide a valuable framework for research (Prideaux, 2002).

There is a move in medical education towards improving the evidence base of education (Stanley and Spencer, 2000; Bligh and Brownell Anderson, 2000) in parallel with the move towards evidence-based medicine. Education has traditionally relied on qualitative studies, using techniques drawn from the social sciences. These are considered to be of less value than quantitative controlled experimental designs. There are problems in introducing more rigorous experimental techniques into education, not least the complex nature of any educational interaction, the difficulty of isolating variables, ethical concerns about randomization and cost. It can be hard adequately to power a trial, effect sizes are small (Albanese, 2000) and the length of medical education means that outcomes require a long follow-up. It is likely that educational research will need a composite approach.

References

Albanese, M. (2000) PBL: why curricula are likely to show little effect on knowledge and skills. *Med Educ* **34**, 729–38.

Bligh, J., and Brownell Anderson, M. (2000) Medical teachers and evidence. *Med Educ* **34**, 162–3.

Kaufman, D., Mann, K., and Jennet, P. (2000) *Teaching and learning in medical education: how theory can inform practice.* Edinburgh: Association for the Study of Medical Education (ASME).

Prideaux, D. (2002) Researching the outcomes of educational interventions: a matter of design. *Br Med J* **324**, 126–7.

Prideaux, D., and Spencer, J. A. (2000) On theory in medical education. *Med Educ* **34**, 888–9.

Stanley, R., and Spencer, J. A. (2000) Assessing the evidence in qualitative medical education research. *Med Educ* **34**, 498–500.

CHAPTER 2
Learning and teaching

Teachers want students to learn, and so it is important for us to have some understanding of how learning happens. In this chapter we will take a basic look at how students learn, how motivation affects learning, and how you can teach effectively by putting some of these ideas into action.

How students learn

As clinicians we know lots of things. For example, we know the causes of acute urinary retention, how to pass a catheter, and how we feel when we see a patient with benign prostatic hypertrophy. Things we know are commonly divided into three '**domains**': knowledge (facts), skills (things you do), and attitudes (opinions which affect the way we behave). In the example above the causes of urinary retention represent knowledge, passing a catheter is a skill, and our feelings about the patient are our attitudes.

We were not born knowing these things, and so must have learned them. However, these different types of knowing are learned and taught in different ways. In the following section we will focus on learning in general, and look at learning in more detail in Chapter 8, which focuses on the different domains individually.

Dealing with information

At a basic level, we learn when we take in new information and add it to our store of information. However, we are all exposed to huge amounts of information every day which we promptly forget. Why does this happen?

Filing information away

Perhaps we did not notice the information at all. In this case it would not even have gone into our short-term memory. Maybe we did notice it, but our short-term memory was full; after all, it can only deal with seven 'chunks' of information at a time. If it did go into our short-term memory, it may not have seemed relevant or interesting and so we did not add it to our long-term memory. Finally, we may have added it to our long-term memory but cannot retrieve it. In all these cases the information is lost for good—we will just have to relearn it.

Retrieving information

Sometimes we can get the information out but it is not usable. You may be able to recite the differential diagnosis of a sensory polyneuropathy, learned parrot-fashion while a medical student, but find that it does not pop into your head when you see a patient with tingling in her toes. You can get at the information in the right situation (probably in an exam when the question says 'List the causes of . . . '), but you cannot use it to solve practical problems. It appears that there are different ways

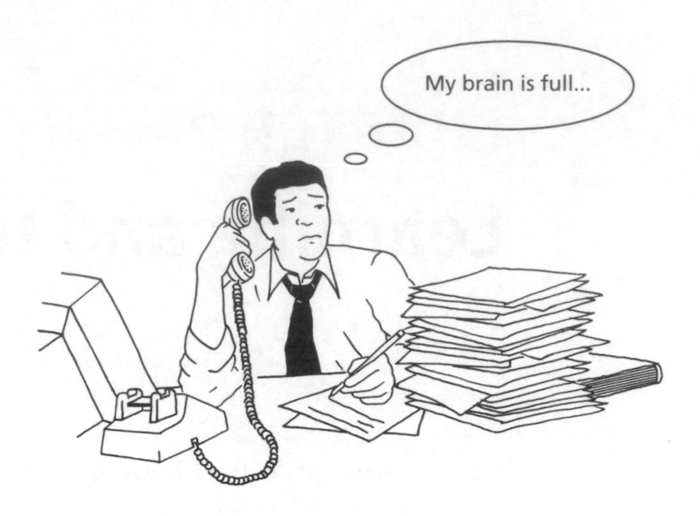

of knowing something—you can recall the facts, you can understand them, or you can use them to solve problems (see Chapter 8 for more information).

What makes some memories accessible and useful? Students sometimes hope that just by dozing in a lecture theatre they will 'take it all in', but failing exams usually teaches them that it isn't that easy: to get something firmly into long-term memory requires work.

How memory works

There are many theories about how memory works, but current evidence shows that information needs to be built on a foundation of pre-existing memory. For this to happen the student needs to identify the previous memory and then build the new information on top in a logical fashion. This information may need moving around a bit in order to make it fit, and to link it to other bits of knowledge. For this to happen the student needs to work with the information. This is very important for teachers, as it underlines the fact that it is not enough for us to impart knowledge—if we want our students to learn, we will have to encourage them to work with the knowledge themselves.

The way in which information passes into the memory has been an interest of psychologists for over a century. There are three broad schools of thought about how students learn, divided into the behaviourists (building on Pavlov's ideas about a stimulus leading to a response), the cognitive school (looking at how information is handled), and the humanists who have examined the innate wish to learn (Curzon, 1994). The cognitive approach, and specifically constructivism (Bruner, 1966; Piaget, 1950; Fosnet, 1996) is currently popular. This posits that learning involves individual transformation, and that individuals actively construct their knowledge out of building blocks of information called schemata. There are several major elements to the learning process: prior knowledge activation, development and modification of schemata, tuning of these schemata, and application of the schemata to problems. By *activating* knowledge they already have, students are ready to start *building* on new knowledge. Once the new knowledge is built onto the old knowledge it can then be *re-ordered* if necessary. By *applying* the new knowledge, the schematas may once more be reordered and the information is then easier to recall in the appropriate setting. The implication of this from the teacher's point of view is that a purely didactic approach will not induce transformation within the learner. For schema construction and elaboration the learner must interact with the information.

Learning in the clinical setting

This seems to apply very neatly to learning from lectures or books, but quite a lot of our learning as students and practitioners takes place in the practical setting. However just experiencing something is not enough to 'learn' it—if that were the case, history wouldn't have a habit of repeating itself. Again it seems we have to work with the new information to get it firmly into our memories. The best way of doing this is to think critically about or '**reflect**' on the experience, develop some ideas about why things went the way they did, and then consider improvements for next time. This is often called the experiential learning cycle (Kolb, 1984).

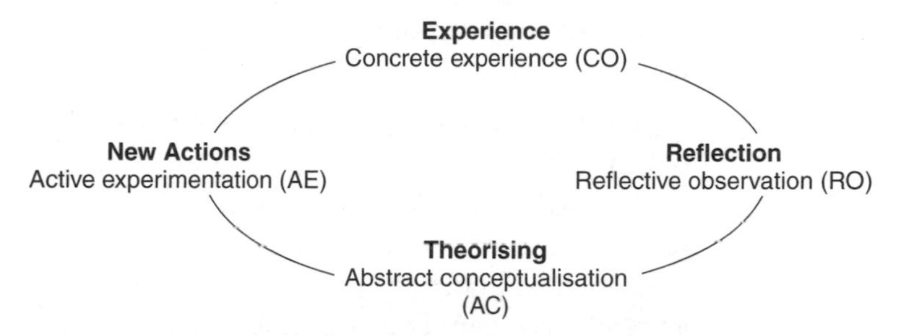

Figure 2.1 The experiential learning cycle (Kolb's learning cycle)

Sometimes we need help with reflecting—someone needs to push us into doing it—perhaps by asking a question, or by giving us some feedback. Feedback may also help us develop new ways with which to deal with the problem next time. This practice–feedback–practice loop is how we learn physical skills.

Kolb's work is developed from the work of Dewey, Lewin, and Piaget, with contributions from humanism, therapeutic psychology, and self-actualization psychology. Kolb describes the cycle as exhibiting two dimensions—that of grasping and that of transformation. The cycle can be drawn to show these:

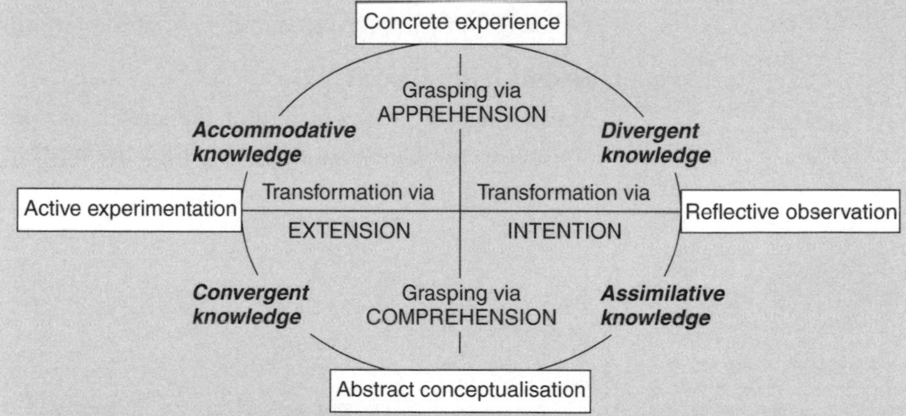

Figure 2.2 The Kolb cycle, drawn to show the two dimensions of grasping and transformation

From this expansion of the basic cycle it is possible to look at different types of knowledge and styles of learning. Other theories of experiential learning also stress the key role of reflection. Schön (Schön, 1987; Argyris and Schön, 1974) proposes that much of our practice is based on 'theories-in-action' (complex sets of propositions that guide behaviour in situations), but that observed behaviour is often due to 'theories-in-use', which are not always congruent with the theory-in-action. Only by reflection on his actions can the practitioner understand his theories and develop them.

Wanting to learn

In order to learn, students need to interact with information. This means we cannot do the learning for them, because if they don't make the effort they won't learn. When faced with a student who isn't learning, we have to ask ourselves whether the problem is that they don't want to learn or whether they can't. The thing that pushes students to learn is called '**motivation**'. Motivation may come from many things—your students may want to learn in order to be good at their jobs, to pass examinations, or to keep up with their peers. They may not want to learn about neuropathy (knowledge), breaking bad news (a skill), or the approach to patients with a substance abuse problem (attitude) unless they understand how it will be useful or whether they are going to be assessed on it.

Studies on motivation have identified two types of motivation (Fry *et al.* 1999). *Extrinsically* motivated students are concerned with getting good grades, external rewards, and approval from classmates, while *intrinsically* motivated students enjoy a challenge, are curious, and want to learn. Within these two types there are different degrees of motivation. Some students are very driven to learn and have been described as having *achievement* motivation (Entwhistle and Ramsden, 1983) while others seem to completely lack any drive to learn, and are referred to as *amotivated*—they perceive themselves to be incompetent, don't know why they are studying, and feel they have little control over what happens to them. There is a link between motivation and *learning strategy* (which refers to the type of learning adopted by the student, covered more fully below), and the combination of motivation and learning approach can predict academic success (Garcia and Pintrich). Thus students who lack intrinsic motivation can still perform well if they adopt appropriate learning strategies.

Being able to learn

Many educationalists think that humans have an innate urge to learn, and in the right environment will do it automatically (Rogers, 1983). If a student wants to learn but isn't able to, we need to ask ourselves what is interfering with the learning process.

Finding it too difficult

Sometimes the problem is that the subject is too difficult. It may be that the student hasn't identified a firm base for the new information, that it is presented

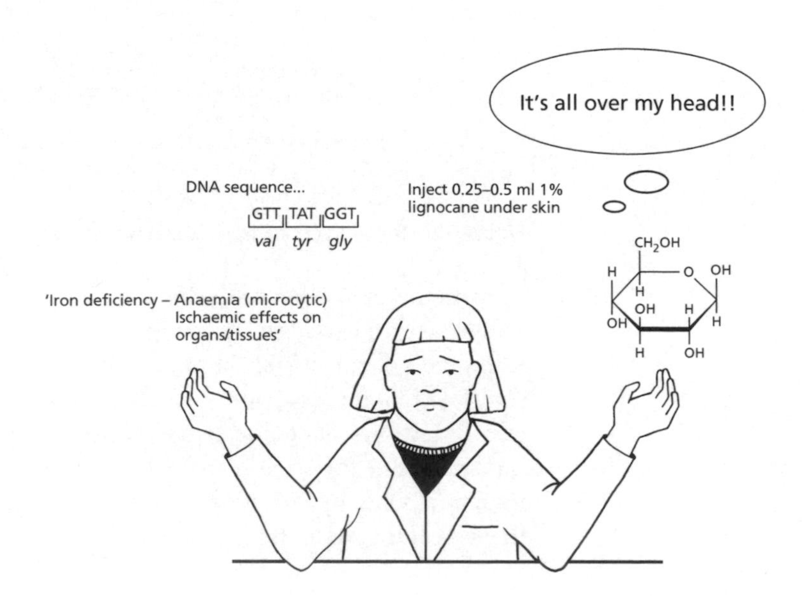

too quickly, or in a way they don't understand. Students learn at different rates and in a group, some may have already incorporated the information, while others just can't catch and integrate the information fast enough.

Being comfortable

Like tender plants which wither at the first touch of frost, students are susceptible to the prevailing '**educational climate**'. You might imagine that this refers to the dreadful chill in many seminar rooms, and it is certainly difficult to learn if you are cold, hungry, or tired (see Chapter 3 on getting organized for teaching). However, apart from the physical environment, the educational climate has emotional and intellectual aspects. It is hard to learn if you are unhappy, worried your tutor may humiliate you, or feel ill at ease with your fellow students (**emotional climate**). On the other hand, no matter how positive you feel, if your teachers and fellow students do not value learning and your contributions are not welcome (**intellectual climate**) you won't be able to learn. Happily most medical students do want to learn, and if the conditions are right they will flourish.

Approaches to learning

Motivated students in the right conditions are ready to learn. However, they don't all approach learning in the same way. In fact there are two distinct approaches. Some students learn by rote, often in order to pass exams, and are described as *surface learners*, while others try to understand the topic and are described as *deep learners*. There is no doubt that deep learners develop durable and useful knowledge, but interestingly may not do as well in some kinds of exams.

A combination of the two is seen in the *strategic approach* where students adopt some techniques from each style in order to pass exams. Students with this learning style seem to do best of all in medical school examinations. While surface learning may well lead to students passing exams, they need to understand that this will not always result in usable information in the future.

Learning styles

If you think about any group of students, it is obvious that they don't all learn in the same way. Some like to take part in active discussions, others like to think things through, or 'have a go' on the wards. Our preferred way of learning is termed our *learning style*.

There are several different classifications of learning styles, and they all come with handy 'find your own learning style' questionnaires. The most commonly used classification was derived by Honey and Mumford, who divide learners as follows:

(a) **Activists**—are open minded, try anything once, thrive on the challenge of new experiences, but get bored quickly, are gregarious, and want to be the centre of attention.

(b) **Pragmatists**—like to try out new ideas to see if they work in practice, act quickly and confidently on ideas that attract them, and are impatient with open-ended discussions. They are down-to-earth, like solving problems, and making practical decisions.

(c) **Theorists**—like to adapt and integrate observations into logical maps and patterns in a step-by-step way. They are perfectionists, detached, analytical and objective, and dislike the flippant or subjective.

(d) **Reflectors**—like to collect lots of information and think about things thoroughly before coming to a conclusion. They are cautious and stand back from meetings, appearing tolerant and unruffled.

A student's approach to learning and learning style is reflected in their *learning strategy*, which is the method of learning they adopt—some students go to the library, others make copious notes, and others like to discuss what they are learning with their peers. None of these is necessarily the 'correct' way to learn, but some strategies are less successful than others. Students may find, to their dismay, that strategies that worked well in the past (for example when revising for A levels) are less successful in undergraduate or professional assessments.

Students like to find out their learning approach and style, and it is useful for them to do so. While the approach and style may not be easy to modify, an experienced teacher or a study skills course can help students select the right learning strategies, and make the most of learning experiences that suit them.

There are many models of learning styles, reflecting the complexity of the topic. Underlying learning styles are preferences in the cognitive processing of information and these are linked to personality traits (Curry, 1983). These influence the way in which learners learn, which then affect the type of learning experience they seek. The concept of learning style attempts to synthesize these factors together, and pick out different types of learner. The three most commonly quoted models of learning styles are those of Honey and Mumford (1992) described above, Kolb (1984), and Pask (1976). The latter looks at how learners like their information presented: *serialists* learn best one step at a time, while *holists* learn from the 'big picture' and fill in the steps later. Kolb's learning styles depend on the degree to which students use each of the four components of the experiential learning cycle. This can be plotted onto the two dimensions of the learning cycle, and the quadrant in which the student is strongest identified. Students tend to come out stronger in one quadrant, giving four basic learning styles—the convergent (problem solvers / decision maker), divergent (lateral thinkers), assimilative (inductive reasoners / theorizers), and accommodative (active risk takers). This contrasts with the approach of Honey and Mumford, whose model also gives four styles, activists, pragmatists, theorists, and reflectors. There is no doubt that the two models give styles that overlap to some extent.

There has been considerable debate about the degree to which learning approaches and styles are modifiable. It is likely that both learning approach and learning style are habituated, and may not be easy to change. These scores seem stable over time, and it is interesting that those in different professions seem to have different learning styles, although whether this reflects selection or education is unclear. The professions (including medicine) tend to be convergers, while the social professions (nursing, teaching, social work) tend to be accommodators.

In summary, students learn by actively building new information on the foundation of previous knowledge. This learning process works best when the student is well motivated and in a supportive environment. Students have different learning approaches and styles, and adopt learning strategies to reflect this.

How teachers teach

What is a good teacher?

Having thought about the basics of how students learn, how do we teach? The aim of teaching is to help students learn, and a good teacher is one who can inspire students to learn to the best of their individual abilities.

All of us can identify teachers who were inspiring, and who helped us to learn something new. What is more difficult is to think why those teachers were good. Sometimes it helps to contrast them with teachers who had the opposite effect on us—whose lessons were endured, and whose legacy put us off their subject forever.

In staff development activities over many years we have asked potential teachers to reflect on what makes teachers good or bad. Their answers always fall into the same categories, and we have used their reflections to describe what they feel are good teachers:

- Good teachers create a good atmosphere in which students feel able to ask questions. They make sure that all the students contribute in a group and take their contributions seriously. They make sure they know what the student needs to know and the level they are at. Because of this their teaching is challenging.
- Good teachers are well organized, and everyone understands what they will learn in a session (the students may even look up information in advance). Their organization extends to having a clear structure to a session, with a summary of the most important points at the end of the session. Because good teachers are well prepared they use good visual aids and may even have handouts.
- Good teachers are enthusiastic and enjoy teaching. Although they may not always keep to time, they don't cancel sessions unexpectedly or are repeatedly late. Their enthusiasm for teaching and their subject is infectious and students therefore turn up on time and participate fully.

This description feels very daunting. Most of us would settle for having just a few of the attributes and, although we want to being inspiring teachers, often fall far short, usually due to circumstances that we feel are outside our control. You might even conclude that wonderful teachers 'are born, not made'. This is not true. Teaching is a skill, and like all skills can be learned.

Teaching as a skill

A skill is rather like a jigsaw puzzle. To learn it you need to break it down into its component parts, figure out what each piece is and where it goes, and then put it together.

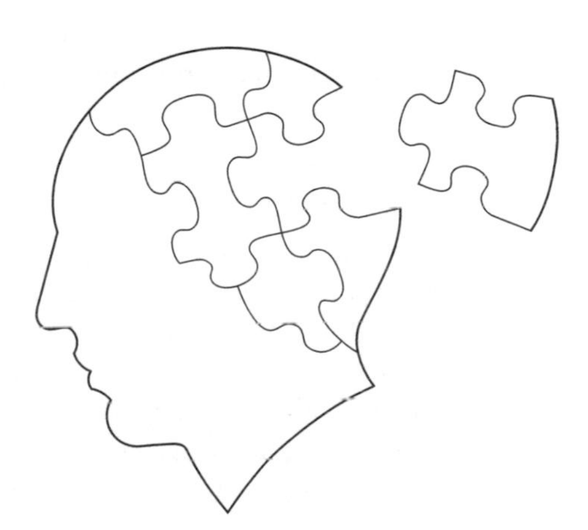

The 'skilled teacher' puzzle has the following three pieces, each of which can be further split up:

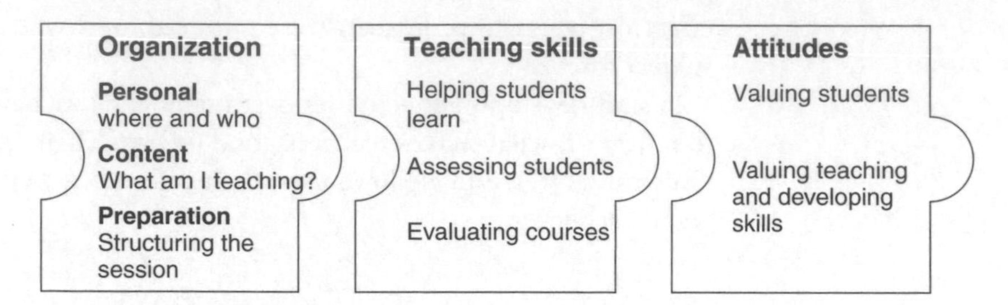

Figure 2.3 'Skilled teacher' puzzle

Organization

Organization is very important, and will be dealt with in more detail in Chapter 3. Not only do you need to be in the right place at the right time, but you also need to know what you are teaching, how, and to whom. You may be familiar with the area, but if you are expected to teach on a new subject, you may need to spend some time understanding new information, and anticipating the sort of questions your students are likely to ask. The preparation of a session is very important, and may take as long or longer than the face-to-face teaching.

Teaching skills

Effective teachers use a battery of techniques to interest their students, teach at the right level, and make the most of their time. We will look at these skills in more detail in Chapter 4 on basic skills for teaching.

We now know that learning is an active process, in which students build information in their brains. Just throwing information at them and expecting it to stick will only work for a minority. To teach effectively, you need to encourage this active learning process, and the following tips are useful:

Encouraging active learning

- Make sure that the environment is right—when the students are comfortable and well motivated, they will be able to learn most efficiently.
- Ensure that students have a firm foundation for new information—they will need to identify things they already know which are relevant. This may be from school, work on the wards, or from their life experience.
- Present the new information in a logical way to make it easier to incorporate.
- Encourage them to work with the knowledge to make it usable, either by discussion or problem solving.

Attitudes for teaching

What attitudes do we need as teachers? This is a difficult area, but one that is very important. Often when teaching goes wrong it is because either the teacher or the students do not want to be there at all. There are lots of reasons for this: for example you might be desperately busy in the clinical side of your job; have family problems; or just have had enough of teaching.

Over the years, as teacher trainers, we have come across very few cases where people who really wanted to teach and be good at it, did not go on to be successful teachers. If you want to be a good teacher and have the time to work at it, you are likely to succeed.

Even if some of the other problems listed above hinder you, you are likely to reorganize your clinical load or persuade someone to give you a hand with your family.

When teaching is too much

At the end of a hectic day of juggling teaching and your clinical load you may well feel that you have had enough of teaching. This is particularly common when you have been teaching on the same programme for years—the challenge has gone, and the teaching is getting a bit boring. If you are feeling a bit like this read the last chapter of this book first. It will help you to focus on the benefits of continuing to develop as a teacher. You might find that changing the teaching programme you are on, learning some new teaching techniques, or even doing a teaching diploma will help you feel much more positive about teaching. However, if you have really had enough of teaching, or the additional workload is overwhelming, think about giving it a rest for a while. A teacher who doesn't want to teach is not likely to teach well. Perhaps someone else in the firm, or one of your partners in practice would like to take it on for a while, and after a few months you may find that you would like to go back.

Being a good teacher

There are many ways to be a good teacher. Teachers are individuals, and use different teaching strategies to teach. Students have different learning styles and teachers have different '*teaching styles*'. Because of this we suit some students better than others. However, a good teacher is flexible, and can adapt to different students. You will find plenty of ideas for teaching in the following chapters. We encourage you to try out as many different teaching techniques as possible, find the ones that suit you best and keep the others in reserve—you never know when you may need them.

Finally, remember that you don't have to be a great showman, a comedian, or intensely charismatic to be a good and highly regarded teacher. In fact when you reflect back on such individuals who taught you, you may remember them warmly but not necessarily remember what they taught you. Their behaviour may have distracted you from learning. A good teacher is enthusiastic, shares their love of the subject and that, together with a firm grasp of the key skills of teaching, is enough.

There has been considerable research into effective teaching at school and university level. Studies have shown that students can clearly and reliably distinguish a good teacher from a good performer, are not fooled by a teacher's popularity, can rate their ability at feedback, and are sensitive to the teachers attitude to teaching and the subject they are teaching. Students identify the important characteristics of teachers as: organization, stimulation of interest, good explanations, empathy, good feedback, clear goals, and encouraging independent thought. Far less important are the teachers personality and sense of humour (Ramsden, 1992). This list correlates closely with lists generated by teachers (Fry *et al.*, 1999; Ramsden, 1992), from which Ramsden has compiled six principles of effective teaching.

1 Interest and explanation.
2 Concern and respect for students and student learning.
3 Appropriate assessment and feedback.
4 Clear goals and intellectual challenge.
5 Independence, control, and active engagement.
6 Learning from students.

Similar lists have been generated within medicine (see Chapter 3).

Conclusion

Students learn by actively building information in their brains. This information needs to be built on a solid foundation and be linked to other information in the right way, so that it is accessible and useful for solving problems. This learning process requires work on the part of the student, and will only happen if the student is motivated and comfortable.

Teachers help students to learn by encouraging this process. To teach effectively requires a combination of good organization, teaching skills, and attitudes, and nearly all of us can learn to be good teachers by developing our skills.

References

Argyris, C., and Schön, D. A. (1974) *Theory in practice: increasing professional effectiveness.* San Francisco: Jossey-Bass Inc.

Bruner, J. (1966) *Towards a theory of instruction.* Cambridge Mass.: Harvard University Press.

Curry, L. (1983) *An organisation of learning styles, theory and constructs,* pp.185–235. London: ERIC.

Curzon, L. B. (1994) *Teaching in further education: an outline of principles and practice,* 4th edn. London: Cassell Education.

Entwhistle, N., and Ramsden, R. (1983) *Understanding student learning.* London: Croom Helm.

Fosnet, C. T. (1996) *Constructivism: theory, perspectives and practice.* New York: Teachers College Press.

Fry, H., Ketteridge, S., and Marshall, S. (1999) *A handbook for teaching and learning in higher education: enhancing academic practice.* London: Kogan Page.

Garcia, T. and Pintrich, P. R. (1996) The effects of autonomy on motivation and performance in the college classroom. *Contemp Educ Psychol* **21**, 477–86.

Honey, P. and Mumford, A. (1992) *The manual of learning styles.* Maidenhead: Peter Honey.

Kolb, D. A. (1984) *Experiential learning—experience as the source of learning and development.* NJ: Englewood Cliffs.

Pask, G. (1976) Learning styles and strategies. *Br J Educ Psychol* **46**, 12–25.

Piaget, J. (1950) *The psychology of intelligence.* London: Routledge and Kegan Paul.

Ramsden, R. (1992) *Learning to teach in higher education.* London: Routledge.

Rogers, C. (1983) *Freedom to learn for the 1980s.* New York: Macmillan College Publishing Co.

Schön, D. A. (1987) *The reflective practitioner.* San Francisco: Jossey-Bass.

CHAPTER 3
Preparing for teaching

To be a good teacher you need to be organized, have the skills to get your message across, and want to teach. Good planning underpins all good teaching sessions, and no matter how skilled, charismatic, or humorous a teacher, if they are repeatedly late, disorganized, or teach postgraduates about the basics of diabetes, students will not turn up and make pointed comments on course evaluation forms.

In the last chapter we looked at how students learn, and the key features of good teachers. This chapter will guide you through the three main organizational steps you need to consider before you actually start teaching; getting organized, sorting out the content of the session, and planning how to deliver your teaching.

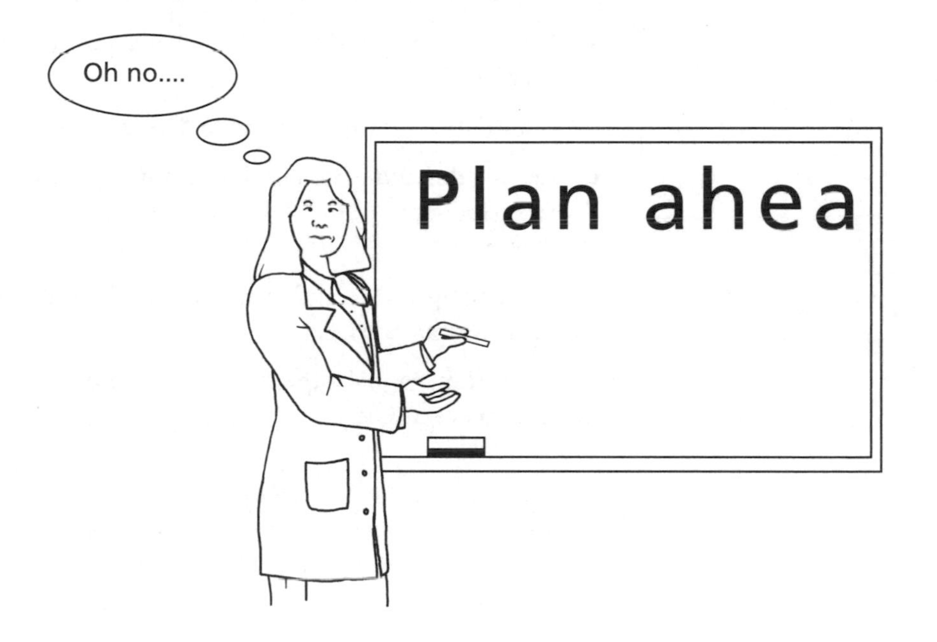

Getting organized

It is important to consider a few basic areas before you actually meet with the students. These may seem straightforward but considering a few fundamentals before you start can avoid problems later. For simplicity we have divided these into four groups; who, where, when, and what am I teaching?

Who am I teaching?

There are three main things to find out. First, you need to know what level the students are at. There is a huge difference between teaching medical students at the start and at the end of their course. You will want to know precisely where they are in the year, where they are in the course, and what experience they have had before.

Secondly, you need to know how big the group is likely to be. You will plan very different teaching for two students, six students, or 30 students. Finally, you will want to know if there is anything particular you should know about any of the students. Some of them may be re-sitting the attachment or having personal problems. Others may be experts in the area, for example mature students with previous experience.

'I was going to teach about nutrition in the elderly, when the group started to laugh. I asked what the problem was and they indicated a mature student who, it turned out, had a degree in nutrition—he was an invaluable resource, and the other students and I learned a lot.'

Where am I teaching?

Making sure you know where you are teaching avoids embarrassing delays while you and the students search for each other. Medical schools are often short of space and use all sorts of odd venues in neglected corners of old buildings. If the venue is totally inappropriate you may be able to get it changed—sometimes for something worse. It is worthwhile getting to know the potential teaching spaces in your medical school and trying to book them far in advance. Check that you can get into the room, and whether you will need any special identification to get access to the building.

It is useful to run through a brief checklist of practicalities.

- Does the room need setting up beforehand, and if so can I do it alone or will I need help?
- Is it suitable for what I intend to do, e.g. small group work or lecture?
- Are all the audio-visual aids (from flip chart paper and pens through to PowerPoint projectors) I want already supplied or do I need to order them? Do they work?
- Is the temperature and ventilation of the room adequate or should I request extra heating/fans?

It is important to make the students as comfortable as possible, as this will help them learn effectively.

Attention to the environment is important for learning. The environment can be thought of as a mixture of physical and psychological factors. These were characterized by Maslow, in his hierarchy of needs (Maslow, 1970), and shown diagrammatically below.

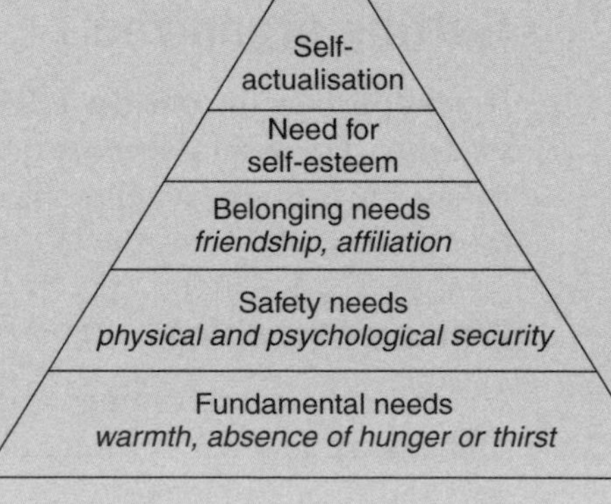

Following this schema, a learner cannot proceed to the next level unless the needs of the previous level have been met. Thus a student cannot learn effectively unless they are comfortable physically and mentally. Ensuring a comfortable environment is a basic organizational issue, while developing an appropriate psychological environment is a key teaching skill.

When am I teaching?

This relates both to your own workload and to the student timetable. Think about when the teaching is occurring in relation to other commitments you may have that day or week. Check your diary to see whether you have other activities going on. These may complement the teaching—students may benefit from coming with you on a domiciliary visit if the patient agrees—or you may have to rearrange things to fit your teaching in. It is unlikely that you can make your clinical work completely disappear, but you may be able to arrange some protected time. Asking a colleague to hold your bleep or be duty doctor for an hour will allow you to teach in relative calm.

It helps to know in advance how your teaching fits into the student timetable, as knowing what they have done will make it easier for you to plan the content of your session (see below). Despite careful timetabling it is common for teaching sessions to clash. It is worth checking with the students that their version of the timetable is the same as yours to avoid problems.

What am I teaching?

Reflecting on what you will be teaching beforehand is fundamental, but particularly when teaching in clinical settings, it is an area that is often missed. We will go on to cover this in more detail, but key questions to ask yourself are:

- *How does the topic fit into the students overall curriculum for the whole attachment*? You may find that they have covered some of the basics already, and that more complex stuff will be in a future course. Knowing this you can tailor the content of your session appropriately.
- *What is this course trying to achieve*? These may include some generic skills (for example communication skills or ethical considerations) as well as those specific to the topic you are teaching. These should be listed in the student course guide. You may spot potential areas of overlap, and it is worth liaising with other course teachers to reduce these.
- *What is my session trying to achieve*? You may be given a list of aims for your session, and you should then plan your session around them, as your students will be assessed on them.
- *How will the students be assessed on the topic I am about to teach*? Assessment is one of the most powerful driving forces for learning. If your topic is not already included in their assessment then consider creating your own assessment as part of the teaching, or to include in their end-of-course examinations (see Chapter 9). The type of examination your students face will lead them to request different types of learning (see Chapter 9).
- *Has anyone taught this topic before*? If so, they may have teaching materials (overhead transparencies, slides, handouts, etc.) that you can use or adapt.
- *Am I prepared for teaching that topic*? You may need to revise or read up on the background to the topic or the latest evidence in that area. It is often helpful

to identify student resources in advance (e.g. a basic textbook, CD-ROM, or web site).

- *Do I need any extra resources*? You may need to find patients, books, anatomical models, or medical equipment.
- *Do I have the appropriate teaching skills*? You may need to speak to more experienced colleagues, read and reflect about the technique, or go on a refresher course to use the teaching methods you will need.

If you have followed all the organizational tips you will know exactly who you are teaching, when and where, and will have a rough idea in your mind of what you are going to cover with the students. Unfortunately a rough idea of the content of your session is not enough to properly plan a session. Good teachers have a precise idea of what they are going to teach, and use this to determine the structure of the session.

Getting the content right

At first glance this is the easy part of teaching—you may be a world expert in your field, and are confident that you can deliver a lecture on balloon valvuloplasty in mitral valve disorders. However your undergraduate students are hoping to see a patient with a murmer and talk about what that noise might mean. Getting the content of the session right for your students is very important.

In many cases you will know (sometimes quite exactly) what you need to cover in the session. At other times it may be up to you to figure out what to cover with your students. If this is the case there are three main steps for you to go through to determine what exactly you are going to teach:

(1) Negotiate what the students want to cover bearing mind what the course covers—its '**aims**'.

(2) Determine what the students need to know in order to meet the aims.

(3) Frame this as a precise statement of what they are going to learn—an '**objective**'.

Aims, objectives, outcomes, and competencies

You are likely to hear the terms '*aims*' and '*objectives*' frequently in your teaching role. In summary, an aim is the broad intention of the teaching programme. An objective is a more detailed statement of exactly what you intend the student to know or be able to do at the end of the programme. This may seem a bit basic, but it makes an important point. Students are likely to learn best if they know what they are setting out to do (the aim) and how they are going to achieve this (the objectives).

A problem faced by medical schools is that the knowledge practicing doctors need to know far exceeds what they can achieve in a curriculum. The traditional subject-led approach (i.e. asking specialists what should be on the curriculum, and then deriving objectives from this) has led to massive factual overload. An alternative is to try to look at what the PRHO or Intern should be able to do at the end of the course. This is called an '*outcomes approach*', and you will come across the terms educational '*outcomes*' and '*competencies*'. An outcome is what you want the student to be able to do eventually— in the case of medicine when they qualify. As you expect that the student will be able to perform to a certain standard (i.e. be competent), they are also called competencies. Competencies are divided into generic competencies (like communication skills) and subject-specific ones (like venesection or managing an MI). They are rather like objectives, but in reverse. When you write objectives you start from a syllabus, whereas with outcomes you start from what you want the finished product to do.

There is a current trend in educational development to focus on your 'end-product' or outcome and the core competencies in your field rather than produce a long list of objectives without any clear idea of the final product you are hoping to achieve (Dunn *et al.*, 1985).

The work of Ramsden (1992) and Entwhistle and Ramsden (1983) supports the need for students to be given some form of aims and objectives in order to gain a clear idea of where they are going and what is expected of them. Objectives are statements with no obvious end-point, and their high degree of specification promotes surface learning (Dent and Harden, 2001). There is a current trend towards 'Outcome-based education' that emphasizes the product rather than the process of medical education (Harden *et al.*, 1999; Prideaux, 2000). There is growing concern about professional competence and reliability within the media, and the reputations of doctors may be seen to depend on the skills of the weakest members of the profession (Eraut, 1994). Recent studies in the United Kingdom have shown that pre-registration house officers (PRHOs) or Interns have significant gaps in their knowledge and skills (Williams *et al.*, 1997; Jones *et al.*, 2001). This needs to be addressed at the undergraduate level by reconsidering core competencies for undergraduate medical curricula (Dunn *et al.*, 1985). The core competencies of a PRHO have been laid out by the GMC in their documents '*The new doctor*' and '*Good professional practice—duties of a doctor*' (General Medical Council, 1998b, 1998a).

Negotiating with the students

Teaching about something the students want to learn is the best way of making sure that they are motivated and will pay attention. In most cases you and the students will have some idea of the aims of the course, which should be provided by your course leader, or the medical school. By checking what they have covered already, you will be able to make a list of things they need to learn. It is often helpful to do this on a flip chart. An ENT teacher might end up with a list that looks something like this:

What we need to learn about ENT

Otitis media	Tonsillitis
Deafness in adults	Hearing aids
Deafness in children	Glue ear
Tinnitus	Cochlear implants
Sinusitis	Vertigo

Looking at this student-generated list and comparing it with the course aims might show that some course aims are completely missing—for example tumours of the head and neck, and that other subjects are listed that could be taught together: for example deafness in children and glue ear.

What you teach at each session depends on how many sessions you have the students for, the resources (patients, models, etc.) available, and the complexity of the different subjects. Together you should be able to prioritize the list, and decide what you are going to teach.

Narrowing down the content

By assessing the students prior knowledge, you can find out what they know already about a topic. As a clinician, you may know that there are certain things that you need to able to know or do first, before you can tackle the topic that the students have chosen. For example if they want to be able to hear the murmur of mitral stenosis, but do not understand how these sounds are produced, you will need to cover that in the session as well to ensure that their new skill is underpinned with the appropriate knowledge. It is possible to represent all the things that your students need to know to understand a topic using a 'concept map', as shown below.

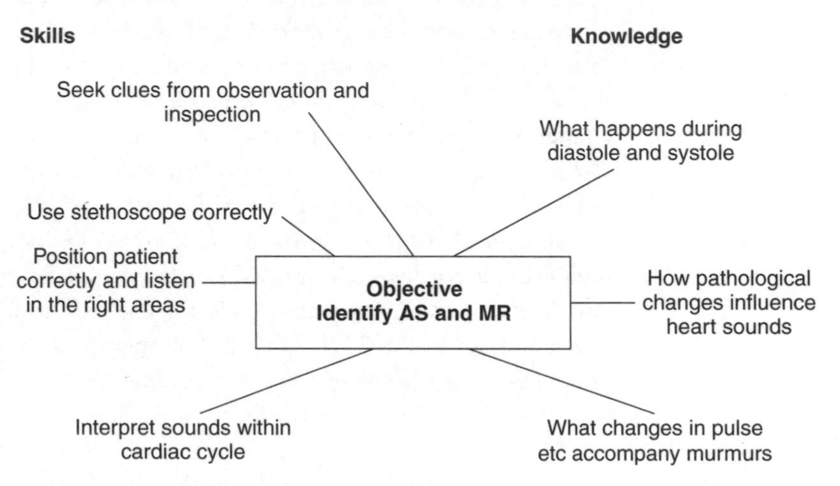

Figure 3.1 Concept map for identifying cardiac murmurs

Getting a clear idea of what the students already know and what they need to know ensures that you do not make the session too complicated or too easy. The level of the content is known as the '**pitch**'. If the content of the session is too difficult then it has been pitched too high. If the session is too easy then it has been pitched too low.

Once you have more idea about what you need to cover in the session, not only what the students want to know, but also what the students need to know, you are ready to start writing it down in the form of objectives or competencies.

Constructivist theories of learning imply that for new information to be incorporated it needs to be built on existing knowledge. If this is absent or inadequate learning will not occur. This implies that some information is required before more can be learned. This is termed a '*learning prerequisite*'. Content can be represented as a hierarchy that places concepts in ascending order. For teachers this has the important implication that concepts should be clearly defined and their interactions understood (Reigeluth *et al.*, 1994). A practical way to investigate this is task analysis or '*concept mapping*', the results of which can be represented diagrammatically.

From a concept map the content structure of the session can be determined. This content structure can be used to determine the learning prerequisites which must be understood for a student to be able to learn something more complex.

Why writing down objectives or competencies is useful

Sitting down and writing either aims, objectives, or the core competencies and outcomes (we're not saying do all four!) for your teaching can really help to focus your mind on what the important 'bottom-line' messages are for the students. It will help you to plan the body or middle of your teaching session, and sort out the 'nice to know' from the 'need to know'. It also helps focus planning or writing questions for assessing students—with a well written objective you can often simply put a question mark on the end and you have a ready-made exam question.

You may find that the objectives are already written. This is useful, as it tells the teachers before and after you what you plan to do. It is still worth checking with the students that they are appropriate, and even if they are well written, you may find it helpful to re-frame them and tailor them to exactly what you intend to teach. If changing objectives, it is important that you stay within the framework of what is required, as otherwise your colleagues may make false assumptions of what the students have covered in your sessions and the students may end up with gaps.

Having a rough list of objectives and competencies is all very well, but to make them really useful they need to be expressed in a way which can be understood by any teacher or student.

The General Medical Council (GMC) in the United Kingdom has stated that the ultimate aim of any medical course should be to train a competent pre-registration house officer or intern (PRHO), who then will go on to have further training in their specialism (General Medical Council, 1993). These PRHOs will need to have skills for lifelong learning but do not need to have specialist level subject knowledge in any given area. Therefore, for most undergraduate teaching, the competencies required are those that a PRHO needs to identify and manage common problems in your subject area. This would include understanding their own limitations and recognizing when they need to seek extra help.

A list of generic competencies can be found in the GMC documents '*The new doctor*' and '*Good professional practice—duties of a doctor*' (General Medical Council, 1998b, 1998a) which can be a good starting point. How you can integrate these into your teaching is covered in more detail in Chapter 8. Subject-specific competencies will obviously vary depending on your field. These have often already been defined, for example by your relevant Royal College. You may find them in the published literature, often in education journals which would be searchable in Medline database using search terms such as 'curriculum'. There are good examples of these for paediatrics and psychiatry (Walton and Gelder, 1999; Haddad *et al.*, 1997). These tend to have quite long exhaustive lists, and an important next stage is to consider what is achievable in the time you have available.

How to write a good objective

Objectives can be written in three areas: knowledge, skills, and attitudes. Knowledge objectives are often the easiest to write. Attitudinal objectives are usually found to be the hardest and so consequently are frequently missed out. For most topics you will be able to write objectives in all three domains.

Some mnemonics have been created to aid remembering the key elements (TIPS, 1976). The first of these is the 'A, B, C, D' of good objectives.

Good objectives should include attention to the following components:

A	*Audience*	Who is it for and what is their level of prior knowledge?
B	*Behaviour*	What should they be able to know/do after the session?
C	*Conditions*	What are the conditions under which you expect them to achieve the objective?
D	*Degree*	What degree of expertise should they have at the end?

For example:

At the end of this session . . . . the third year clinical medical students with no prior training (A) should be able to insert a foley catheter using an aseptic technique (B) on a skills model (C) without assistance on two out of three attempts (D).

In the second, good objectives should 'RUMBA'.

R	*Relevance*	Relevant to the students learning needs.
U	*Understandable*	Written using plain language, short sentences, and a new objective for each different component.
M	*Measurable*	With content that is testable in assessments—adding a question mark on the end of the statement should turn it into an exam question.
B	*Behavioural*	Identifies some form of change (in knowledge, skills, or attitudes) in the students.
A	*Achievable*	Realistic for the student to achieve at the given level with the conditions, teaching methods, and available time.

Below are some examples of good and bad objectives from an obstetrics and gynaecology attachment defined using 'RUMBA'.

'*Students should be aware of the importance of examining the abdomen in normal pregnancy, in particular determining the fundal height, foetal lie, and foetal heart rate.*'

This objective is not very well written. It was actually intended for new fourth year medical students, but as this is not stated you might think that it could be applied to a postgraduate audience who would feel it was rather basic. It seems understandable on first reading it, but in actual fact it is rather vague about what the students can actually expect to learn in the session. It is difficult to measure an 'awareness' accurately, and no actual behaviour change has been stated. Taken out of context it is difficult to know if it is achievable.

'*By the end of this session, fourth year medical students in week one of their attachment will be able to:*

- *demonstrate a complete abdominal examination of a woman with a normal pregnancy in the third trimester including:*
- *measuring the fundal height*
- *locating the foetal lie*
- *eliciting the foetal heart rate using a sonic-aid device*'

This is a well written objective. It seems highly relevant to fourth year medical students, and is understandable as it has been broken down into simple component parts which would be easy to teach. It would be easy to measure and test as part of a clinical examination, documents clearly the new skill or behaviour the student is expected to acquire, and seems likely to be achievable in the context given.

Writing good competencies and outcomes

Very similar rules apply to writing good competencies and outcomes. The key thing to remember is that rather than working forward from the syllabus, you are working backwards from what you want the students to be able to do at the end. It helps to start with the outcomes, with a clear idea in mind of exactly what the junior doctor should have to do. Outcomes are rather like aims: they state in broad terms what the students should be able to do. Competencies can be framed more like objectives, but are usually less precise.

Once you have re-framed what the students want to learn in objective and/or competency form, you will have a list that looks like the one below.
Two ways of presenting the content of a community-based session on attitudes to mental health for third year medical students.

Aims and objectives

Aims

To understand what it is like to live with a mental health problem in the community.

Objectives

Describe the experience of illness of two patients or carers who have/have recovered from different mental health problems (depression/anxiety/adjustment reaction, alcohol/substance misuse) in primary care.

Consider the potential impact a diagnosis of a mental health problem could have on an individual.

Discuss how patients interpretation of mental health symptoms influences their health behaviour and interaction with medical care.

Outcomes and competencies

Competencies

Understanding the influence of psychological symptoms on health behaviour and interaction with medical care.

Understanding of what it is like to live with a mental illness including social stigmatization.

Outcomes

Students who can:

Communicate effectively with patients with psychological problems.

Understand the problems faced by patients with psychological problems.

View the presentation of psychological problems in a holistic way, understanding the complexity of presentations to health care professionals.

Common problems with objectives

Many people struggle to write objectives and often find that the ones they write are either too vague or are too detailed and expect too much from the students. It is difficult to move away from broad terms such as 'be aware of' or 'understand' which are hard to measure or test. It helps to use certain verbs which are more precise.

Verbs which describe behaviour for use to aid writing objectives:

Knowledge	name	classify	describe	contrast	evaluate
	state	identify	compare	distinguish	solve
	list	outline	define	differentiate	assess
				explain	collate
					calculate
Skill	demonstrate	show	establish	formulate	assemble
	elicit	make	present	summarize	modify
	measure	operate	illustrate	organize	maintain
	locate	use/utilize			apply
Attitudes	recommend	defend	challenge	judge	persuade
	adopt	advocate	argue	justify	question
	select	debate	contest	advise	
	suggest	assert	specify	consider	

People also complain that objectives often lack context and that it is impossible to write an objective for every part of the curriculum that students need to learn. In fact the problem is more to do with factual overload in the medical curriculum and the recognition that it is not possible to include everything. One of the core tasks of lesson planning is deciding what bits to leave out. Writing and reviewing your set of objectives (making sure they are 'Achievable') is one way of tackling this.

No matter how perfect your aims and objectives are, if the session is poorly structured, the students will not be able to make sense of any of the information. The next step is to plan how you will structure your content to ensure that the students learn as efficiently as possible.

Structuring your session

'Tell 'em what you are going to tell 'em, tell 'em, and then tell 'em what you have just told 'em.'

Anon

Getting the structure of your session right will help your students learn. Although in the short-term it may appear a time-consuming task for a busy clinician, in the long-term it is likely to save you time. The first time you plan a lesson it will take a long time. However you will become quicker with practice, and the use of a lesson plan enables you to store your preparation for future sessions.

Planning, organization, and structure have for many years been reported as one of the key attributes to effective teaching and learning (Irby, 1978; Metcalfe and Matharu, 1995). The process of structuring a session is informed by the principles of '*instructional design*'.

Several influential theories of instructional design have been developed, but the most frequently used is Gagné's model (Gagné *et al.*, 1988). This is based on an information processing model of learning, and can be criticized from a constructivist standpoint. However it is still widely used because it provides a systematic way to approach teaching. There are nine stages.

1 Gaining attention.
2 Informing the learner of the objective.
3 Stimulating recall of prerequisite learning.
4 Presenting the stimulus material.
5 Providing learning guidance.
6 Eliciting performance.
7 Providing feedback about learning.
8 Assessing performance.
9 Enhancing retention and transfer.

Within a session, structuring techniques used by successful teachers include *signposts* (statements signalling the direction and structure), *frames* (delineating beginning and end of topics and sub-topics), *foci* (highlighting key points), and *links* (statements linking sections to each other or other knowledge/experience) (Brown, 1982).

We advocate the use of a simplified model of instructional design, focusing on the three main parts of a session: the introduction, body, and close.

How should I structure my session?

Feedback from students over the years has given us a very clear idea of the structure that they find most helpful for learning. They like teachers to give sessions a clear beginning, middle, and end (or introduction, body, and closure). Good teachers structure each of these three parts in a way that enhances student learning.

Structuring the introduction to your session

The introduction to a session is crucial as it is *the* time when you have the maximum attention of your students. There are five basic elements to a good introduction which we have summarized into a mnemonic to act as an aide memoir—you can 'MMOPP' the floor before you start by considering the *M*ood, *M*otivation, *O*bjectives, *P*rogramme, and *P*rior knowledge.

Mood

Setting the right mood from the beginning is very important. It is set within the first few moments of a session, so capitalize on this by immediately making the students feel welcome and at ease. Starting a session by chastising students who are late or the AV technician because there is no slide projector gets everyone off to a bad start. Check that there are no burning issues that the students would like to discuss first. If it is your first session with a group, it is worthwhile informally discussing some ground rules, covering issues like attendance and confidentiality (see Chapter 5).

Motivation

Motivate the students to learn by explaining how relevant the skills learnt will be for them both as medical students and doctors, whatever their specialty. Remember that for students, assessment is a powerful driving force (see Chapter 10). A good way to motivate the students is to describe a time when your learning of this topic has been useful to you in practice. Try and choose a scenario that the students themselves are likely to face in the near future. It is no use telling first years 'this will be useful when you are on call'. Personalizing the learning is an important motivator.

Objectives

Give students a clear idea of the learning outcomes and how they are going to achieve them by sharing your aims and objectives. Sharing the aims and objectives helps both you and the learner focus on the task in hand, and will help you check towards the end of the session whether you are on track to meet all the objectives.

Find out the student's learning needs and check that these match your objectives. They may have other learning needs that they would like you to address, or would like you to focus on some particular topics or skills. Often the objectives need to be negotiated with the students at this stage. You may need to slightly alter the objectives you have prepared to match the needs of the students and make the session truly 'student centred'.

Programme

Show students that you have carefully planned the session, and let them know what is going to happen by outlining a basic programme for the session they are about to have. Tell them how this fits into to their overall learning programme. Students don't like surprises, and need to know about course content and timing in advance in order to plan their learning. Students benefit from knowing how the new learning fits in with what has come before and what is coming next. This allows them to activate the prior knowledge that they will need to start learning new information.

Prior knowledge

Find out what students already know about the topic first. This helps to pitch the session at the right level and also allow them to identify the foundations on which they will be able to build new information and link new knowledge and existing knowledge together. Activating this old knowledge in students' minds at the start helps them to make these links.

Checking prior knowledge is not the same as asking about students confidence in a given area, which may not be directly linked to their actual competence. Likewise simply asking about attendance at previous teaching sessions on the topic will not necessarily give you an idea of what was actually learnt and retained by the students. It is worth probing a little to find out exactly what they know.

Having started your session off using a MMOPP, you will have relaxed students who are keen to learn, know exactly what they are going to cover in the session, and have activated the prior knowledge they need to start building on new information. How do you structure the body of your session to ensure that they learn efficiently?

Structuring the 'body' of your session

Getting your students to build usable memories requires you to feed them structured information, and get them to interact with it. To do this they will need to be awake, remain interested, and participate in the session. If you are covering several objectives it is helpful to signpost clearly when you are moving to a new topic, link it in to other topics, and clearly highlight the key points in a mini summary before moving on to the next topic. This technique will help you to control the rate at which you deliver the content. This rate is called the '**pace**'. Good teachers keep the pace of a session quick enough to ensure that students are challenged, but not so fast that slower students are left behind.

Some useful tips to consider when planning the main part of any teaching session are considered below.

Less is more

Most teachers have a tendency to try and cram in as much as they can in the session to 'cover' the topic. Students will actually learn more if you have less content, feel less rushed, and have opportunities to reflect and discuss key areas. In general only three or four new concepts can be properly covered in one sitting. Look critically at your objectives and divide them into 'need to know' and 'nice to know'. Thinking about what you would highlight in the summary at the end will help you to pick out the 'need to know' points. Try to jettison some of the 'nice to know' content—it may only end up confusing the issue.

Vary the stimulus

We can only concentrate on a passive task for a short time. A lot of medical school teaching is passive, and a lot of students lose concentration.

Human beings seem to be able to pay close attention for very short periods of time, following which attention falls off. We have an attention span of about 15 minutes, but we rarely have teaching sessions that last only 15 minutes. If you change the content or the teaching techniques you can re-attract the students attention. This new attention span also decays, and you will need to keep changing to maintain your students attention.

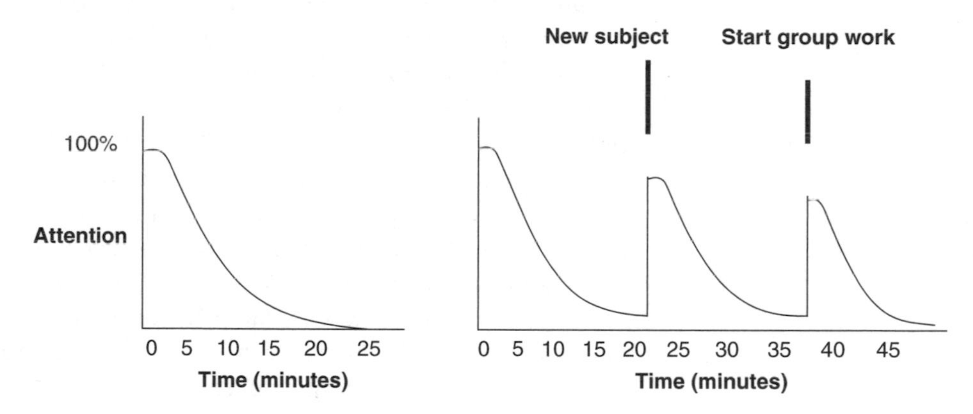

Figure 3.2 Graph of attention span with time

It is therefore helpful when planning to break your session down into 15 minute chunks, and make sure you change the pace or teaching method for each 'chunk' or simply have a break. You can vary the stimulus by changing to a different audio-visual aid, stopping talking and asking for questions, or using one of the techniques for promoting interaction described in Chapter 4 on basic skills for teaching.

Promote interaction

Try to promote interaction from your students, both with you and with each other. This is known as '**active learning**'. This will increase their processing and hence long-term retention of new knowledge, maintain their interest, and is a useful way of varying the stimulus. The various ways of promoting interaction are discussed in greater depth in Chapter 4. When you are working out the timing of a session, remember that an interactive session takes longer than a didactic formal lecture. As a rough guide a highly interactive session will take twice the amount of time to cover the same ground as in a didactic lecture. In a very interactive session you will therefore be able to cover far less content, although what you do cover will be in greater depth and with increased understanding. You may want to balance your session with components of each style. When you are planning, try and work out how much time you have for each activity and note that down. If you overrun on one activity and know how long the others will take you can negotiate with the students which areas to miss out.

Go from the specific to the general

Students find it hard to learn general concepts without having examples in their mind of what you are talking about. For example, students may find it difficult understanding the principles of fluid balance without first discussing this around a case example (either a real one they've seen or a hypothetical case). We look at this more in Chapter 7. Thinking about a case first helps students to identify the appropriate foundations on which they will build the new information, and puts it in context. Once students have engaged with a case or specific situation they will be ready to start drawing out general principles from this.

We recommend that in most cases you start with a specific example and then fill in the information around this. An exception to this is when you have a lot of ground to cover, particularly at the beginning of a course. In this case start off by talking generally about the area, to give students a map of where they are going.

Choose teaching methods to satisfy all types of learning styles

Students vary in the way they like to learn. Different learning styles are discussed in Chapter 2. If you are teaching one to one, you will be able to adopt an appropriate teaching strategy (as discussed in Chapter 4), but within any group you will have a variety of learning styles. This means including practical activities for the 'activists' and 'pragmatists', and integrating time for reflection for the 'reflectors' and 'theorists'. Teachers are likely to choose teaching methods that suit their own learning style. Therefore, if you are an activist or pragmatist, you may fill your session with a series of practical engaging tasks for the students to complete, but not relate these to the underpinning theory or allow adequate time for reflection. Although you can't please all the people all the time, at the planning stage try to ensure that you have elements that will appeal to at least some of your students some of the time. Changing teaching strategy within the session has the added advantage of maintaining your students' attention.

There is substantial evidence to suggest that overloading the students with information encourages students to take a surface approach to learning, rather than a deep approach which has in turn been associated with less long-term retention of knowledge (Marton and Saljo, 1976; Pask, 1976; Entwhistle and Ramsden, 1983; McManus *et al.*, 1998).

Varying the stimulus is important as research dating back to World War II has shown that human attention span tails off significantly after 15 minutes. It has been reported that if there is mismatch between the learning style and the educational environment and teaching style then students performance may be negatively affected (Curry, 1983). Evidence suggests that summarizing and linking new information both within the topic and to external experiences helps recall and understanding and yet is an area that is often missed (Brown, 1982). Theories of professional learning emphasize the importance of learning by experience, reflecting on this experience, and then applying new insights gained into practice in cyclical process (Kolb, 1984; Schön, 1987).

Once you have planned the body of your session, making sure that it is not overloaded with objectives, that the chunks of information are logically ordered and linked to each other, and that you have a variety of tasks to maintain attention and engage your students, you are ready to consider how you will end the session.

Structuring the end of your session

Closing a session properly is important as it capitalizes on a well established brief increase in attention from the student to reinforce your key messages. It can also provide students with a sense of achievement which itself has been linked with better long-term retention of knowledge. There are five main elements to a good closure. The 'LASTT' things you have to do before you leave are to: Leave out questions, Achievement, Summarize, Think (for students), and Think (yourself).

Leave out questions

Questions are very important to a session, but should be kept within the body of the session. By ending your session with 'Any questions?' you risk your students remembering the questions rather than your vital take home messages. Time should be left to clear up any questions *before* you commence closing the session; you might otherwise get distracted on some small point rather than reinforcing their learning of key points. Students tend to remember the last things they experience more so use this time to drive home your key learning points.

Achievement

Provide students with a sense of achievement—this will aid their further motivation and learning. This can be done by assessing whether they've learnt anything by a short quiz or by returning to the objectives and asking them to recap the key points. Even a simple statement that they have worked hard or you are pleased with their input or effort can give a 'feel good' factor that will aid learning.

> *'OK we set out at the beginning of the session aiming to get you all suturing correctly and I have seen each one of you produce a near perfect stitch: well done!'*

Summarize

Students, like patients, tend to remember the last thing that you say to them, so make sure that your message is clear and concise. A summary at the end of a session will help your students to identify and retain the most useful information. This repetition of key information will aid transfer into long-term memory. It works even better if you can get the students themselves to summarize the key learning points. You can do this by asking them to tell you the key points or to write them down and discuss with their neighbour to check they have all recognized them.

Think—for the student

Encourage the students to apply the newly acquired skills and knowledge in practice. Something that is not practiced or repeated within the next 24 hours is soon forgotten. You can also encourage them to make links between this new learning and either past or coming sessions.

Think—for the teacher

Give yourself a few minutes to reflect on how the teaching has gone. What went well? Is there anything you would do differently next time? Try to briefly jot down a few comments on your teaching plan (see below)—this may be invaluable when asked to teach again in the future.

Having thought through your session in detail, you have a clear idea of exactly what you plan to cover in each section. The problem with all your good ideas is remembering them. The human memory has limits, and in the heat of a teaching session you may be unable to recall what you planned to teach next. Having an aide memoire in front of you is enormously reassuring, but how can you distil all that you have planned into a portable form?

The teaching plan

A teaching plan is a simple written method of planning what you will cover in advance. Using a teaching plan you will be able to see at a glance how much time you can allocate to each bit of a topic, what extra equipment you will need, and what areas you may like to read over beforehand. Within the session it is invaluable to help you keep to time, or to see at a glance what you can miss out if you have been side-tracked. You may find it useful to highlight in your teaching plan the core bits you don't want to miss out, and identify areas or tasks you can omit if you are running out of time.

The actual structure of a teaching plan could not be simpler. Photocopy these two pages onto a sheet of A4 paper. Use the front (marked 'Teaching plan') to note down how you plan to deliver the session, and the back to reflect on the session afterwards. Keeping your old teaching plans is very helpful: not only are they a great resource when you have to teach the session again—cutting down your preparation time enormously—but they should also go into your teaching portfolio as proof of the quality of sessions that you have delivered.

Teaching plan

Subject: **Date:**

Objectives:

	Time	Content	Exercises and resources
Introduction			
Body			
Summary			

Reflection

What went well and why?

What was less successful and why?

What would I change next time (objectives, structure, etc.)?

Extra resources / preparation that would be helpful

Successful teachers often plan their sessions directly onto the teaching plan. This allows you to make sure that there is enough time for everything. Using your list of objectives and the teaching method you have chosen for each part of the session you can write down the time at which you will start each activity, what you will cover, and what resources you will need. A teaching plan may go through several drafts before you are happy with it. An actual teaching plan is shown below.

Teaching plan

Subject: Heart sounds **Date:** 08/09/01

Objectives: Describe anatomy and physiology of the heart, list common causes of valve damage, and identify the murmur of mitral regurgitation.

	Time	Content	Exercises and resources
Introduction	14.00	• Check they are all comfortable, and that there are no 'burning issues'. • Introduce content and objectives. • Have they heard any murmurs yet and do they know what they heard and why? (checking prior knowledge)	• Present case of Mrs F, to show why knowing about murmurs is important and remind them that they are common short cases in finals.
Body	14.15	• Go over anatomy. • Look at relevant physiology. • Look at what damages heart valves.	• Use diagram of heart. • Get students to explain cardiac cycle and normal heart sounds.
	14.25	• Get students to think how this could affect blood flow.	• Picture of stenotic valve.
	14.30	• How does damage affect heart sounds? • Learning to pick out changes in heart sounds.	• Use diagrams in textbook. • Use CD of heart sounds and phonocardiograms.
	14.50	• What symptoms might arise in valvular disease? • What questions would we want to ask in a history?	• Get students to think logically (causes and haemodynamic effects). • Brainstorm list onto flip chart and order it.
	15.00	• Introduce patient (Mrs A with AS). • Discuss findings.	• Get students to take a history and then examine her in turn. • Students to draw what they heard and make diagnosis.
	15.40		• Re-examine Mrs A as necessary.
Summary	15.50	• Summarize important points. • Remind them: diabetes next week.	• Get each one to say what they learned from the session. • Give handout.

Once your teaching plan has been finally written down, you are ready to teach. Do not despair if it has taken you hours to prepare your first teaching session. The best teachers put a lot of time into preparation, and it is common to spend four or five times as long as the actual session in preparation. For large lectures on subjects you don't know well, you will need longer than this. However, not only will you get quicker with practice, but if you save your teaching plan and reflection, next time you teach the same session, your preparation will be much shorter.

Practical tips on good lesson planning

- You can probably only cover three objectives well in a one hour session—so try to limit yourself to roughly these proportions.
- Divide the content you want to include into 'need to know' and 'nice to know'.
- Omit most of the 'nice to know' sections, adhering to the principle that 'less is more'.
- Highlight on your lesson plan the essential 'need to know' sections. If you find you are running out of time when you actually teach the session, or have been diverted then you can easily re-focus yourself onto the core components of the topic. The bits that are not highlighted can be jettisoned or left for another time.
- When allocating how much time to spend on each component of your teaching, allocate time for your introduction and closure first as otherwise these are often forgotten.
- You can then divide the remaining time you have into roughly 15 minute 'chunks' with a different activity for each 'chunk'.
- Immediately after you teach the session complete the reflection section so you know what changes to make when you teach the topic again.
- File your plan somewhere accessible—you may find this invaluable when called on to teach at the last minute in the future.

Conclusion

Good planning and preparation are vital for effective learning and teaching. There are three areas to consider before teaching—organizational aspects, the content of your teaching, and the structure of your session.

Remember to check various organization aspects, asking yourself who, where, when, and what am I teaching? Then think about the content of what you are teaching, and narrow this down to some clear objectives (or competencies), which are realistic, understandable, measurable, behavioural, and achievable. Next, structure your session with a clear introduction, middle, and end. Within the introduction aim for a motivating start that clearly demonstrates the structure and direction of the session. For the middle section, aim to cover three objectives and maintain attention, and improve learning by integrating interaction and different learning methods. Make sure you leave time for a concise closure, repeating key messages to enhance learning and encouraging students to reflect and apply the newly acquired knowledge, skills, or attitudes further. Finally keep a record of your planning using a teaching plan, in order to help you in the session and save time in the future.

References

Brown, G. (1982) Two days on explaining and lecturing. *Stud Higher Educ* **2**, 93–104.

Curry, L. (1983) *An organisation of learning styles, theory and constructs*, pp.185–235. London: ERIC.

Dent, J. A., and Harden, R. (2001) *A practical guide for medical teachers.* Edinburgh: Churchill Livingstone.

Dunn, W. R., Hamilton, D. D., and Harden, R. M. (1985) Techniques for identifying competencies needed of doctors. *Med Teach* **1**, 15–25.

Entwhistle, N., and Ramsden, R. (1983) *Understanding student learning.* London: Croom Helm.

Eraut, M. (1994) *Developing professional knowledge and competence.* London: Falmer Press.

Gagné, R., Briggs, L., and Wager, W. (1988) *Principles of instructional design*, 3rd edn. New York: Holt, Rinehart and Winston.

General Medical Council. (1993) *Tomorrow's doctors. Recommendations on undergraduate medical education.* London: General Medical Council.

General Medical Council. (1998a) *Good medical practice.* London: General Medical Practice.

General Medical Council. (1998b) *The new doctor.* London: General Medical Council.

Haddad, D., Robertson, K. J., Cockburn, F., Helms, P., McIntosh, N., and Olver, R. E. (1997) What is core? Guidelines for the core curriculum in paediatrics. *Med Educ* **31**, 354–8.

Harden, R., Crosby, J., and Davies, M. H. (1999) *AMEE medical education guide No 14: Outcome-based education.* Dundee: AMEE.

Irby, D. M. (1978) Clinical teacher effectiveness in medicine. *J Med Educ* **53**, 808–815.

Jones, A., McArdle, P. J., and O'Neill, P. A. (2001) How well prepared are graduates for the role of pre-registration house officer? A comparison of the perceptions of new graduates and educational supervisors. *Med Educ* **35**, 579–85.

Kolb, D. A. (1984) *Experiential learning—experience as the source of learning and development.* NJ: Englewood Cliffs.

Marton, F. and Saljo, R. (1976) On qualitative differences in learning. *Br J Educ Psychol* **46**, 4–11.

Maslow, A. H. (1970) *Motivation and personality*, 2nd edn. London: Harper and Row.

McManus, I. C., Richards, P., Winder, B. C., and Sproston, K. A. (1998) Clinical experience, performance in final examinations, and learning style in medical students: prospective study. *Br Med J* **316**, 345–50.

Metcalfe, D. H., and Matharu, M. (1995) Students' perception of good and bad teaching: report of a critical incident study. *Med Educ* **29**, 193–7.

Pask, G. (1976) Learning styles and strategies. *Br J Educ Psychol* **46**, 12–25.

Prideaux, D. (2000) The emperor's new clothes: from objectives to outcomes. *Med Educ* **34**, 168–9.

Ramsden, R. (1992) *Learning to teach in higher education.* London: Routledge.

Reigeluth, C. M., Merril, M. D., and Bunderson, C. V. (1994) The structure of subject matter content and its instructional design implications. In *Instructional design theory* (ed. M. D. Merril and D. G. Mitchell). Englewood Cliffs: Educational technology publications.

Schön, D. A. (1987) *The reflective practitioner.* San Francisco: Jossey-Bass.

TIPS: *Teaching improvement project system.* (1976) USA: The Kellogg Foundation.

Walton, H. and Gelder, M. (1999) Core curriculum in psychiatry for medical students. *Med Educ* **33**, 204–11.

Williams, C., Milton, J., Strickland, P., Ardagh-Walter, N., Knapp, J., Wilson, S., *et al.* (1997) Impact of medical school teaching on preregistration house officers' confidence in assessing and managing psychological morbidity: three centre study. *Br Med J* **315**, 917–8.

CHAPTER 4
Basic teaching skills

Once you have prepared your session and made a teaching plan you are ready to teach. Most of your preparation will have focused on the **content** of what you plan to teach, and the teaching methods you will use. However, to deliver a good teaching session you need to get both the content and the **process** of teaching right. Just as you can learn to plan the content of a session, so you can learn the basic teaching skills used by all teachers. These skills can be thought of as a 'toolkit'. You will need every one of the skills during a teaching session. Initially you may find using the different skills rather uncomfortable. However, as you practise teaching you will be able to select the right skill without thinking about it.

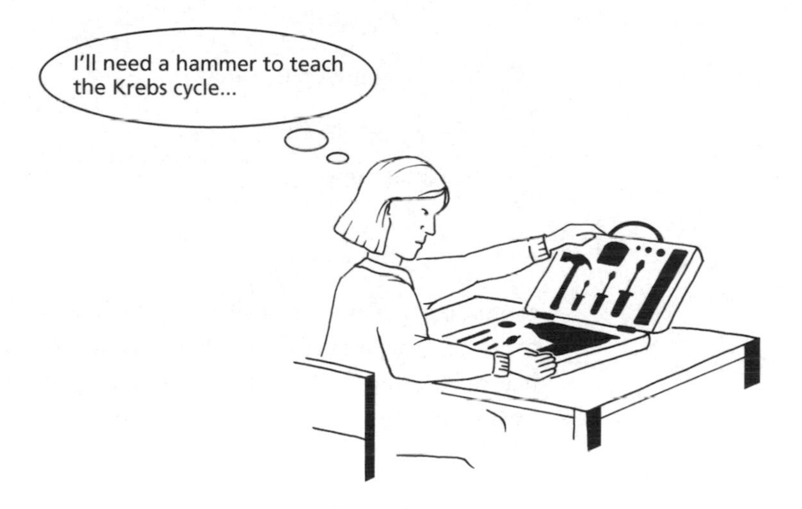

Many of you are already teaching using the skills described in this chapter without necessarily being conscious of doing so. However, to develop these skills further you need to be aware of what you are doing so that you reflect on your teaching and increase your effectiveness as a teacher.

The teacher's toolkit shown below contains the basic skills that you need to deliver any session, anywhere. However, some forms of teaching need specialized skills, and these are described in Chapters 6–8.

Setting the scene

Physical factors

As discussed in Chapter 2, the physical environment of any teaching session is important. Students cannot learn if they are too hot or too cold or if they cannot see a demonstration or hear a tutor. Many medical schools have a shortage of

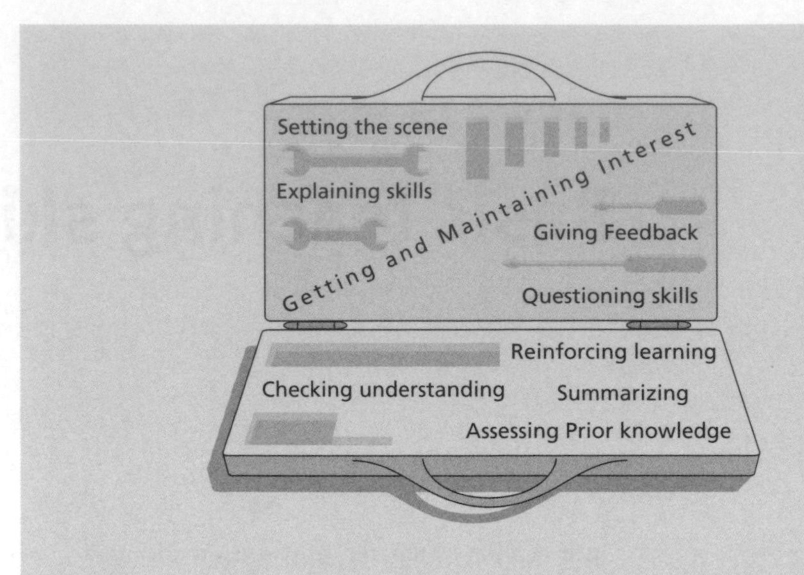

Teachers educational toolkit

1 Setting the scene.
2 Getting and maintaining interest.
3 Assessing prior knowledge.
4 Explaining skills.
5 Questioning skills.
6 Giving feedback.
7 Checking understanding.
8 Reinforcing learning.
9 Summarizing.

rooms, particularly for small group teaching, and must use accommodation intended for other purposes such as laboratory work. It is worthwhile checking out a room before you start—if it is really unsuitable you may be able to find another one or at least adapt your teaching to the environment.

If you are providing individual opportunistic teaching in a hospital corridor you could move to a suitable site where you can talk freely without being asked to move out of the way or being overheard.

A common physical factor disrupting teaching is the interruption of sessions by 'phone calls or bleeps. Try and organize protected time away from your clinical work. Not only will you feel more relaxed, but you will be able to concentrate and follow your lesson plan. Ask your students to switch off their mobile phones—their personal calls are very disruptive.

A small group session taking place in a large lecture theatre with fixed rows of seating will run very differently from the same group taught in a comfortable room with participants sitting in a circle. A circular or horseshoe arrangement of chairs has advantages for both students and teachers. The student can see and hear the tutor or facilitator easily and the tutor can maintain eye contact with all the students, monitoring how the lesson is going by observing the students' body language. A circular arrangement feels more 'democratic' than rows of chairs as all seating positions are of equal importance and the tutor as part of the circle becomes closer in status to the other group members. Teaching around a table may be more convenient for writing but can also act as a barrier between teacher and students.

Getting the scene right also includes checking that all your instructional materials, handouts, etc. are available, that the IT is working, and you know where to find the electric plugs and light switches. Arriving early to check physical arrangements and to move furniture is good practice and allows you to start the teaching session as soon as the students arrive.

Setting the scene

Physical factors

- Check heat, light, and seating.
- Check audio-visual aids are working.
- Arrange the furniture.
- Minimize interruptions.

Psychological factors

- Welcome students.
- Set ground rules together.
- Make it clear that you respect and value their contributions.
- Use a facilitative style.
- Encourage questions.

Psychological scene setting

Going to a party where the music is live loud jazz will induce a very different mood from a party which welcomes you with a classical quartet. We can stimulate a mood conducive to learning in various ways. If the room is already set up, the teacher calm and welcoming with a notice or overhead displaying the title of the session, then the student will feel reassured that they are expected and in the right room. Informal chatting to the first arrivals serves the dual purpose of showing your willingness to engage with students and checking their expectations or prior knowledge.

Most teachers have vivid memories of themselves or colleagues being taught 'by humiliation'. Enquiries about such experiences invoke passionate responses about incidents that happened years earlier, reviving the unpleasant feelings of the time rather than the facts the teacher was trying to instil. Unfortunately this type of teaching still occurs occasionally. A more effective method of encouraging learning is to ensure that students feel safe to express ignorance or doubt and are valued as a group and as individuals. We can encourage students to express their uncertainties, but if they feel that their colleagues are going to belittle their efforts, they will be unwilling to open up. One way round this is to set ground rules which are agreed by all students. These should include listening to everyone with equal attention, and encouraging questions, however basic. The right '**educational climate**' is very important for effective learning and creating a suitable educational climate is one of the key tasks of a teacher. Allowing or encouraging a certain amount of informality can enable your students to relax.

Your teaching style, which depends on your personality and experience, will be reflected in the educational climate you offer your students. You need to make sure that you cater for students' varying learning styles and adjust the teaching for each style. You can do this in several ways including:

(a) *Matching*—you can try to match your teaching style to the students learning style.

(b) *Choice*—provide several forms of learning within a session or course; ask the students what they would prefer.

(c) *Guided independent study*—let the students study using their preferred learning strategy using materials which have been prepared for them.

In practice we often don't know our students' learning styles, making matching difficult. So it may be wise to offer a choice of different learning methods within each session or series of sessions. It is helpful to mix small group learning and large group learning, offer students the chance to try practical tasks as well as reflect on material they have seen, and offer handouts from lectures containing guidance on further reading. You could ask students directly how they would prefer to work. This approach will cater for a wide variety of learning styles.

The existence of different learning styles is not in doubt and their relationship to cognitive processing and learning strategy is beginning to be understood (Curry, 1983). The classifications of learning style are discussed in Chapter 1. Honey and Mumford's learning styles can be extrapolated to activities that suit different learning styles.

Activists: learn best with new experiences where they can 'have a go', situations where they can be centre stage (leading discussions), brainstorming ideas, and moving from activity to activity. Quick-moving small group work suits them best.

Reflectors: benefit from watching and thinking about activities. They like to carry out research first, review evidence, write careful reports, and need time in teaching sessions to think. They may have a passive role in small group work, preferring to play the role of an observer.

Theorists: like plans, maps, and models to describe what is going on. Enjoy being intellectually stretched by complex problems, but need time to explore methodology, structured learning situations, and a defined purpose. May like small group work and lectures, as long as well organized.

Pragmatists: respond to clear links between subject and clinical work. They like practical problems and are keen to try things straight away, preferably with feedback. They often enjoy bedside teaching.

Motivating students

Getting interest

When planning your lesson you should consider how to attract your students' attention (see Chapter 3). You will want to motivate your students by giving them good reasons why they should pay attention. It is a sad but true fact that the most effective motivating force for students is the assessment for each course or year. We hope that the assessments in your institution are carefully planned to reflect what is required from each course. If this is the case then the course curriculum will appeal to the students, as they will be working with the curriculum in mind and should be interested in your subject matter. If the assessments are not planned ideally then you may need other means to attract interest.

To be motivated, students need to know what they are going to learn. If you discuss your aims and objectives with the students at the start of a learning session and are prepared to negotiate changes to suit the students then they will feel more involved with the lesson and more interested. Remember to limit changes to those that are appropriate to the course or session.

At the beginning of the final two hour session on practising clinical skills with a GP in her surgery, four third-year clinical students requested that the GP should cover the cardiovascular, peripheral, and central nervous system as well as the locomotor system. The GP had planned to cover the peripheral nervous system only and knew that their request would be impossible to fulfil in two hours. She negotiated with the students that they would concentrate on those systems that were most important to the students in the forthcoming OSCE and changed the teaching plan accordingly. This negotiation meant that the students were interested in the lesson as it related directly to their wishes and the GP was satisfied as the original teaching plan was modified in a realistic fashion.

Knowing *what* they are going to learn is not enough: students also need to know *why* they are learning something. They need to know that information will be useful for them to understand current clinical problems, or to help them in their future work. They need to know the context in which to place their new knowledge or skills. Moving from the specific to the general by giving examples often catches students' interest. Consider relating a personal experience with patients, then using the incident to broaden out into the underlying general principles. Putting information into a clinical context may also help students use it more easily in the future.

Maintaining interest

Some teachers have no trouble in keeping students' attention. If you observe their lessons they use a variety of techniques which keep students alert and interested. They combine good presentation skills, involving students in their lessons and an ability to change tack if they sense that the students have had enough. This 'student centred' approach to teaching is a good way not only to maintain interest, but also to maximize learning.

Some tips to help you maintain student interest are:

Active learning—involve the students in the sessions by making them think about the subject.

- Use quizzes, buzz groups, discussion in pairs or triads.
- Ask students to summarize, construct theories, and present results of their discussions.
- Use questioning skills to probe knowledge and get students to think.
- Give students a task to do during the session (e.g. role play, solving a problem, or practising a skill).

Presentation skills.

- Vary pitch and pace of speaking voice and projection of your voice.
- Distributing questions widely around the room will keep students alert in case they are asked to contribute.
- Use eye contact to involve all students. Look around the group as you talk, and remember to include the student sitting on either side of you.
- Use 'signposting' to signal that you are about to start a new section of the lesson. This will enable students to be mentally prepared for the next topic.

Monitor student responses.

- Be aware of students' interest by noting their body language and move to the next part of the lesson plan if they are bored. Planning an activity every 15 minutes will prevent the loss of interest that occurs as attention drops.

Students respond positively to enthusiasm in a teacher, so if you are enthusiastic about your subject share your feeling with your students. There is no need to be charismatic, humorous, or a great showman as students will respond to enthusiastic teachers of all types.

The move to student centred teaching is associated with the work of Knowles (1983), who theorized that adult learning (andragogy) is different from the way in which children learn (pedagogy). While his theories lack empirical evidence, they have been very influential in higher education and have led to the development of related theories of experiential learning (Kolb, 1984) and self-directed learning.

The five key principles of adult learning are:

1. Adults are more self-directed.
2. The experiences they have accumulated help them to learn.
3. Adults are driven to learn only when they feel a need to know something.
4. Adults tend to learn in a problem-based way.
5. Adults rely on internal motivation to drive learning.

As individuals mature during adolescence they move into the pattern of adult learning. This maturation can be hindered by overuse of pedagogical approaches in adolescence (Knowles *et al.*, 1998). Thus students who have come from very didactic school environments can have problems engaging with courses designed using adult learning theory.

Assessing prior knowledge

It is essential to know how much the students already know about the topic of the session. Teaching students about a topic they already understand is boring for them, and teaching a topic that is entirely new may mean that you make the content of the session too complicated. As well as paying attention to the place of your session in the curriculum and the brief for your teaching from the course organizer, it is wise to check students' knowledge at the beginning of each session. Checking what they already know is a powerful way to activate their prior knowledge of a subject, enabling them to start building new information on a firm foundation.

The simplest way of ascertaining students' knowledge is to ask them directly about it. You may uncover a wide range of knowledge within a group and may need to adapt your lesson plan to this. You may also uncover experience without knowledge or knowledge without understanding. A student may declare that s/he knows how to check a patient's blood pressure and has done so on many occasions. Probing questions might reveal that this student has no knowledge of the underlying principles of blood pressure measurement, has experience only with one type of machine, does not know about causes of errors, or the use of blood pressure measurement in context. In this case the student will need further work on the basic principles to ensure that the previous knowledge is fully understood. On the other hand, your questions may reveal that the student indeed does have a firm grasp of all the principles. In either case you may need to adapt your teaching to your students' needs.

Assessing prior knowledge

Why

- Essential for each session.
- Activates prior knowledge.
- Enables right pitch.

How

- Ask students directly.
- Reports from other teachers.
- Consider experience versus knowledge.
- Knowledge versus understanding.

Explaining skills

Getting your information across clearly is important for a teacher. Students value teachers who can explain a difficult concept clearly. How do these teachers do it? First, they have a very clear understanding of the subject themselves. They know what the student needs to know to understand the new information and will check their prior knowledge to make sure that it is adequate. Secondly, they divide the new information into logical chunks and explain it bit by bit. Finally, they use clear language and explain new words and concepts as they go along.

Three approaches to giving an explanation

1. **Interpretive**—this defines the central meaning of a term or statement, e.g. 'Homeostasis means . . . . . . '
2. **Descriptive**—this describes processes, structures, or procedures e.g. 'The nephron works as follows . . . . '
3. **Reason-giving**—this involves giving principles or generalizations, motives, obligations, or values, e.g. 'The current attitude to haemodialysis seems to stem from . . . . '

Students learn in different ways, and may not all understand the same explanation. You may have to try a different approach so that students who failed to understand the first time can grasp things next time. Students may fail to understand for the following reasons:

Language. A number of medical students every year do not speak English as their first language. They are often brilliant students but a proportion of them have difficulties with communication, particularly with colloquial English. It is worthwhile bearing this in mind, and adapting your speech to their needs. Consider talking more slowly, making sure that the students can see your face easily, using a limited vocabulary, and allowing plenty of pauses to check understanding.

Words. Being a native English speaker does not mean that students are familiar with medicine's specialized vocabulary. When a new word or abbreviation appears, the student not only doesn't know what it means, but also loses their train of thought and may miss the rest of the explanation. We further confuse things by using common words in a specialized way, and sometimes rather imprecisely. Phrases such as 'His failure meant he lost his exercise tolerance' are clear to clinicians, but mysterious to students and the lay-public alike. Not only do students wonder what 'failure' might mean, but they miss the inference—perfectly clear to practicing clinicians—that the failure referred to is more likely to be cardiac than renal. You can either explain every difficult word as it comes up, write down words which might cause problems and clarify them at the start, or get students to note down unknown words and define them at the end.

Grammar. English grammar is complex and confusing. We are all encouraged to write clearly and simply, but occasionally forget that long sentences with numerous subclauses are also difficult to understand when they are spoken. It is useful to keep sentences short and pithy. Restating complex phrases is useful, as well as allowing students to rephrase concepts in their own words.

Context. When explaining something make sure that the students are thinking about the same area of medicine. Using a clinical example, discussing aims and objectives, using an advance organizer, and probing prior knowledge are all ways of getting the context clear. Students who come in late to a lecture or seminar often fail to grasp what is going on. This is because they have not understood the context of the discussion. If they had been there at the start, they would have activated their relevant prior knowledge of the topic and started to build the new information on top.

Questioning

Teachers questions

A teacher's questions can be used to reveal the extent of a student's factual knowledge, to encourage a student to display understanding, or to stimulate a student to interact with new information and formulate her/his own theories about a particular topic. Questions can be helpful in monitoring how the session is proceeding and in checking that you have achieved your lesson objectives. They can be used in assessing students and in evaluating your teaching. The way you ask questions contributes to your teaching style and the educational climate you engender. Skilful use of questions is one of the most useful components of the teachers educational toolkit.

The easiest questions to ask are those that demonstrate whether a student knows a fact or not. However, this is of limited use. It tells us whether the student can recall the information, but it doesn't give us any information about whether they understand the fact, or can use it to solve problems. You can probe the level of a student's understanding by carefully phrased questions such as 'How do you think that works?', 'Why does that happen?', or 'What do you think would happen if . . . . . . ?'

The idea that a fact can be known at different cognitive levels was proposed by Bloom, who also divided learning into three domains (Bloom, 1956). The domains of learning were originally entitled the cognitive domain, the psychomotor domain, and the affective domain. They are now often referred to as knowledge, skills, and attitudes. Within the cognitive domain, a taxonomy stratifies knowledge into different levels, with the simple recall of facts at the base of the pyramid.

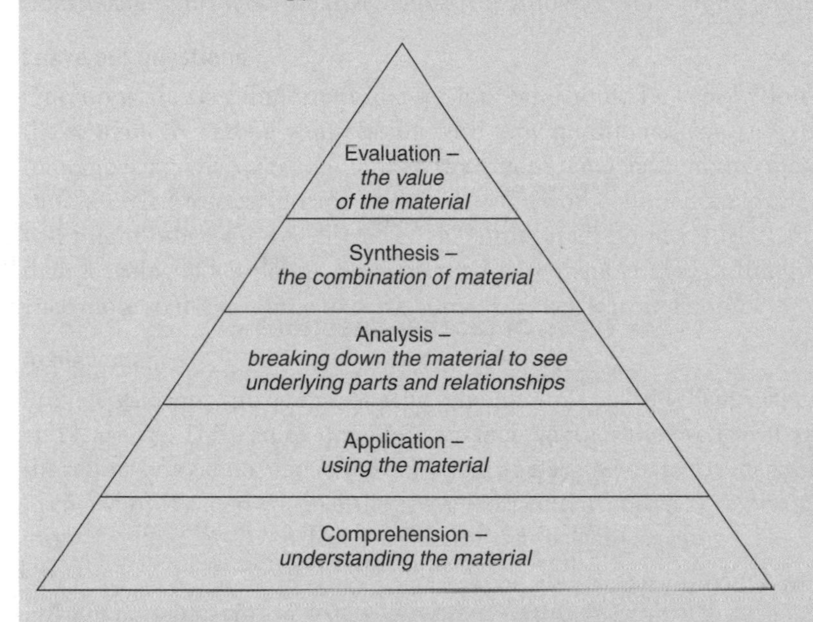

Figure 4.1 The stratification of knowledge into different cognitive levels

Gagné (1985) proposed an alternative model comprising five domains or 'cognitive outcomes': intellectual skills, verbal information, cognitive strategies, motor skills, and attitudes. The category of intellectual skills approximates to Bloom's cognitive domain, and proposes five subcategories: discrimination (recognizing things), concrete concepts, defined concepts (what it is and what it isn't), roles, and problem solving.

The aim of teaching is to move students up towards higher levels of knowledge. Developing higher levels of knowledge takes time, and if students are under pressure to learn a large body of knowledge they are likely to resort to learning techniques which permit them to regurgitate facts without understanding them. This has led to repeated calls for a reduction in curriculum overload from medical bodies nationally (General Medical Council, 1993) and internationally.

Teachers frequently do not allow enough time for students to consider an answer—the more complex or deeper a question the longer a student needs to construct an answer. Teachers often answer their own questions or leave questions unanswered. This gives a sense of incompleteness to the lesson and excludes students from feeling valued as well as indicating to students that questions don't *need* to be answered. Repeating an unanswered question will not produce an answer if the students do not understand the question. Try rephrasing the question or replacing it by a simpler question on the same topic.

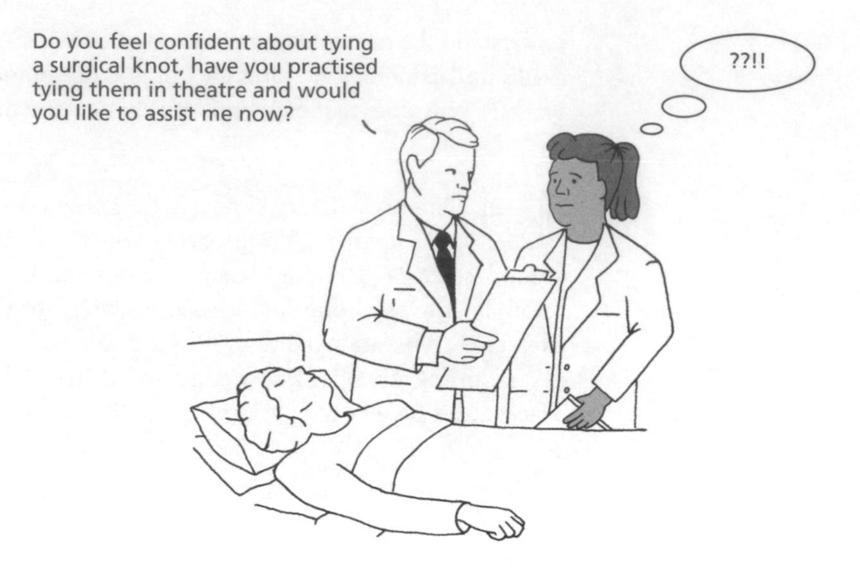

Beware of posing questions with more than one part. As illustrated above, the student might say 'No', 'Yes', or a qualified 'Yes' but as the question was tripartite you will not know to which part a student is referring if they answer 'Yes'.

Types of teacher questions

Another way of looking at questioning skills describes the types of questions you can use. Students and GP registrars will be familiar with open and closed questions from their communication skills sessions. Questions are commonly described as closed or open.

(a) Closed questions (e.g. What are the causes of . . . ?) require a factual straightforward answer without demonstrating ability to put the knowledge to use.

(b) Open questions (e.g. 'Tell me about . . . . ? What do you think . . . . ?) encourage students to think around a topic, to provide imaginative solutions, and to consider complex problems.

As open questions require the student to interact with the knowledge they have rather than just recalling a fact, they are more likely to promote learning.

Student questions

The ratio of teachers questions to students question is said to be 100:1. If you want students to ask you questions you need to attend to the whole atmosphere (the educational climate) of the session. You must also allow enough time for questions and answers. Students can get very adept at distracting teachers from the main topic of a lesson, leading their teachers down interesting but not necessarily relevant pathways. Your lesson plan should be useful in these circumstances by focusing on the main objectives for the lesson and in reminding you of time constraints.

Build in time for questioning throughout your session rather than inviting questions at the end. This keeps students alert. An immediate (or as soon as is practicable) response to a question is more satisfactory for a student while his/her thoughts are concentrated on the topic.

Giving feedback

The aim of feedback is to improve students' performance. If students are upset by the manner in which feedback is offered then they will not be in a psychological state to benefit from it. Students prefer constructive, specific, and immediate feedback that is addressed to their answer or performance rather than as a criticism of themselves personally. There are a number of recognized schemes for giving feedback (Pendleton *et al.*, 1984; Chambers and Wall, 2000) that are used extensively in medical teaching. The box below summarizes the authors' practice which draws on these schemes.

Giving feedback

1 Give feedback as soon as possible after the event.

2 Let the student comment on his performance first.

3 Teacher/observers comment second.

4 Positive feedback before negative feedback.

5 Use specific examples (consider noting them down during the performance).

6 Criticism should be constructive (e.g. suggestions for change).

Feedback needs to be given in a positive spirit in a supportive environment. Focusing on what the student did well shows the level of performance you expect, as well as helping them relax. It is important to be specific about feedback. Vague comments such as 'It was great' are much less useful than 'I really liked the way in which you asked about rectal bleeding because it was an open question'. Cite examples wherever possible—noting examples of good or poor performance and quoting them verbatim is more useful for the students than generalizations.

It is important to give feedback as soon as possible after the event as this keeps the moment fresh in the student's mind. However, when feeding back on the performance of a skill, wait until the student has finished. Continually breaking in to give feedback inhibits learning, perhaps because it disrupts the student's train of thought. Once the student has finished their performance it is tempting to launch directly into giving your own views. Let the student comment on their performance first. This gives you an idea of their degree of insight and helps you keep your feedback centred on their needs.

Student peers are acute observers and with a bit of training can give highly effective feedback. The feedback process will need to be carefully managed by you, and it is wise to remind them of the way in which you would like feedback to be given before each session.

Unfortunately many clinicians behaviour is still modelled on past experience when 'teaching by humiliation' was fairly common. It is not an effective strategy—learning is inhibited by the uncomfortable feeling of humiliation induced by being ridiculed. Even teachers who avoid negative feedback models rarely give positive feedback beyond a simple 'Good' or 'Well done' so missing the opportunity to reinforce desirable behaviour in our students. Making the time to give feedback to students is one of the most valuable ways you can facilitate learning.

There has been considerable criticism of the quality of teaching in medical schools nationally and internationally. Medical school teaching is criticized for its lack of continuity, variable quality, poor supervision, and minimal feedback (Irby, 1995; Metcalfe and Matharu, 1995). The effects of sarcasm and humiliation on medical students and doctors in training continue to cause concern (Lowry, 1992). Several reviews have looked in detail at the need to improve teaching in hospitals, and promoted staff development (Lowry, 1993; SCOPME, 1998; Dearing, 1997). The importance of providing constructive feedback has been repeatedly highlighted.

Students and doctors in training value constructive feedback highly, and have identified it as the most important component of teacher training (Wall and McAleer, 2000). There is evidence that learning is improved by constructive feedback, both in the field of skills learning (Patrick, 1992), and more widely (Rolfe and McPherson, 1995). Feedback improves learning outcomes, develops competence, and helps students adopt a deep approach to learning.

Checking understanding

Checking understanding means making sure that the students understand what you have just covered. You need to know if the lesson is going according to plan so you can continue exactly as in the lesson plan or modify it in line with the students' responses. In checking students' understanding you will automatically be reinforcing their learning.

A clinical lecturer had given the same lecture for ten years to the clinical introductory course students. When the medical school introduced student evaluation of individual lectures he was surprised to find himself rated very poorly for content and delivery. 'But they always say they understand and they are happy' he protested. Further enquiry elicited that the clinician had proceeded to read his lecture as usual and after 50 minutes had looked up from his notes to ask the whole audience if they understood and were happy. Of course they responded 'Yes' to the bipartite question as they did not want to prolong their time in the lecture theatre. Students told the evaluation team that they had not understood the topic from the very beginning of the session and that this was worse for them than the lecturer's delivery.

So how do you make sure that students have really understood? Asking if they understand is not enough—you will need students to demonstrate understanding. If you are teaching a skill you could ask for a demonstration of the skill. A tougher test would be for students to teach each other the skill; in order to teach a skill you need to know how to perform it yourself. During a teaching session you can ask students to summarize after each section or set problems based on the material you have just covered. Asking students to apply their new knowledge in real or invented clinical cases is particularly useful as it sets new learning in a clinical context.

Demonstrating to students that they have made progress is very motivating. Consider setting a quiz at the beginning of a session and at the end set the same quiz. This will serve the dual purpose of motivating the students and checking that they have understood the new material. You could get the students to mark their own or each others answers, or do it as a class activity.

Reinforcing learning

To make the most of the learning they have done in your session, you should encourage your students to continue learning after the session is finished. This should enable them to keep working with the information you have given them, develop links with other information, learn new (related) information, and start to use the information in the clinical context. There are many ways to encourage students to continue to learn, but some useful techniques are shown below.

Teachers who are enthusiastic about their subject, and show that they continue to learn themselves, encourage students to read around the subject. It is important to show that you value students' efforts to learn more. A key point is always to check homework, case studies, or presentations that you have asked your students to prepare.

Reinforcing learning

- Recommend further reading.
- Set written questions.
- Set a clinical problem for students to solve.
- Ask students to clerk a relevant patient on the wards and present them to you.
- Ask students to prepare a presentation on the subject.

Summarizing and closing a session

It is essential to summarize at the end of a session in order to provide a sense of achievement and to reinforce your key points. It is a useful exercise to ask the students to summarize your key messages or to explain how they will integrate new knowledge into future activities, as you will learn how much of your lesson has been noted and absorbed. Do not introduce new material or invite questions at this point in a session—this interferes with a proper sense of closure. You might want to refer to your initial aims and objectives for the session and discuss with the students the extent to which they have been achieved. Just before the end of a session provide an 'advance organizer' for the next session so students can prepare for the next topic. This could take the form of a session title, a paper to be read, or anatomy revision in preparation for clinical skills teaching.

Make it clear when the session is over—close the session firmly with a clear statement and do not let it just fade away.

Conclusion

The 'teachers toolkit' contains a core group of skills that all teachers will need in every teaching situation. Like all skills, these teaching skills will greatly improve with practice.

As an experienced teacher, being aware of the techniques you use when teaching will help you to reflect and improve your teaching performance. This focus on the process as well as on the content of your teaching is valuable for all teachers and will help student learning.

References

Bloom, B. S. (1956) *Taxonomy of educational objectives 1. Cognitive domain.* New York: David McKay.

Chambers, R., and Wall, R. (2000) *Teaching made easy.* Abingdon: Radcliffe Medical Press.

Curry, L. (1983) *An organisation of learning styles, theory and constructs,* pp.185–235. London: ERIC.

Dearing, R. (1997) *Report of the national committee of enquiry into higher education.* London: HMSO.

Gagné, R. (1985) *The conditions of learning*, 4th edn. New York: Holt, Rinehart and Winston.

General Medical Council. (1993) *Tomorrow's doctors. Recommendations on undergraduate medical education.* General Medical Council, London.

Irby, D. M. (1995) Teaching and learning in ambulatory care settings: a thematic review of the literature. *Acad Med* **70**, 898–931.

Knowles, M. (1983) Androgogy: an emerging technology for adult education. In *Adult learning and education* (ed. M. Tight). London: Croom Helm.

Knowles, M., Holton, E. F., and Swanson, R. A. (1998) *The adult learner*, 5th edn. Houston, Texas: Guf Publishing Company.

Kolb, D. A. (1984) *Experiential learning—experience as the source of learning and development.* NJ: Englewood Cliffs.

Lowry, S. (1992) What's wrong with medical education in Britain? *Br Med J* **305**, 1277–80.

Lowry, S. (1993) Teaching the teachers. *Br Med J* **306**, 127–30.

Metcalfe, D. H., and Matharu, M. (1995) Students' perceptions of good and bad teaching: report of a critical incidence study. *Med Educ* **29**, 193–7.

Patrick, J. (1992) *Training, research and practice.* London: Academic Press.

Pendleton, D., Schofield, T., Tate, P., and Havelock, P. (1984) *The consultation: an approach to teaching and learning.* Oxford: Oxford University Press.

Rolfe, I. and McPherson, J. (1995) Formative assessment: how am I doing? *Lancet* **345**, 837–9.

SCOPME (1998) *An enquiry into mentoring: supporting doctors and dentists at work.* London: Standing Committee on Medical and Dental Education.

Wall, D., and McAleer, S. (2000) Teaching the consultant teachers: identifying the core content. *Med Educ* **34**, 131–8.

CHAPTER 5
Content of session

I hear and I forget, I see and I remember, I do and I understand

Old Chinese proverb

The way in which you approach planning and teaching a session depends not only on the group size and setting but also on the content of the session. If you want students to learn how to use an otoscope, they will need to be able to try out the skill. However if you want them to know how to treat otitis media, you might use a less 'hands-on' approach. A good understanding of how students learn knowledge, skills, and attitudes helps effective teachers to tailor their teaching methods to the type of information they are trying to get across.

General principles

The general principles discussed in Chapters 2–4 are key to teaching and underpin all the methods discussed here. Your students will not be able to learn effectively unless they are motivated, understand what and why they are learning, and are comfortable. You will not be able to teach them effectively unless you have clear objectives, have prepared the session, and have some basic teaching skills in your 'toolkit'.

Learning knowledge

Learning new information

When medical students talk about 'knowledge' they often see it as a series of facts, which have to be learned and regurgitated in an assessment. They complain that there is too much to learn, and that a lot of it is irrelevant. For example a student may decide to 'learn all about' atrial fibrillation. He is just starting a cardiology firm and knows that it is likely to come up. Quickly scanning a short textbook he decides that it would be useful to learn the following lists:

The list of things to learn (especially for the first and last items) is very long, but by staying up half the night he commits them to memory. On the ward the next morning he clerks a fit patient with lone AF who has come in as a day case for

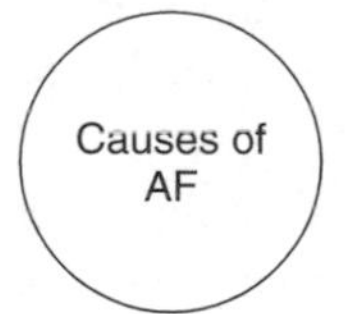

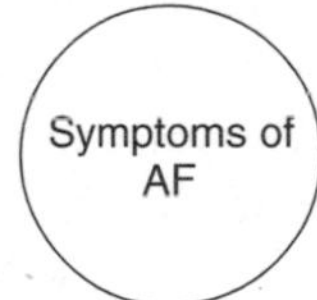

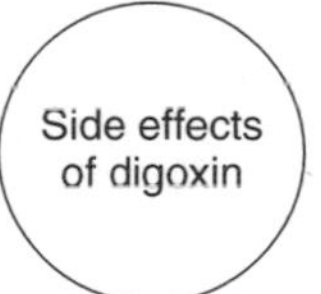

cardio-version. Everything he learned last night seems completely useless, and on the ward round he realizes that he has already forgotten quite a lot of it.

Why has this happened? Our student was well motivated, and prepared to stay up half the night with his lists. Despite this his knowledge was not much use, and he forgot a lot of it. We call this type of learning 'surface learning', and finding difficulties in applying knowledge learned in this way is common.

As clinicians we know that the things he chose to learn are far from 'all about' AF. Unfortunately he didn't know much about AF to start with—we might say he didn't have a clear '**concept**' of it. This would have helped him to understand what AF is, and more importantly what it isn't. If he had done, he might have chosen different things to learn, and developed an understanding of the '**principles**' underlying AF. Building onto knowledge you have already makes assimilation of new material easier, and helps it to be used. If our student had reflected on what he knew about related conditions (perhaps he had a lecture on cardiac arrythmias a week ago) he could then start to build onto this.

Retrieving information

Given that the content of his knowledge was inadequate, why couldn't he use what he had learned? There are several reasons for this. First, in the busy clinical setting knowledge learned in the quiet of the library is hard to recall. If we sat our student down in a quiet corner and asked him to write short answer questions on 'The side-effects of digoxin' and 'The causes of AF' he would probably do pretty well. This is why he has chosen this learning strategy; it worked well at school, where this is exactly the sort of assessment he faced. The problem he now faces is that it doesn't work in the clinical setting. This is because knowledge is often best recalled in the context in which it was learned. It might have been more helpful to see a patient first and then read up in the library after the ward round. Secondly, he has not worked with the knowledge to understand how it fits together. The knowledge currently exists as three isolated lists of facts. If they were interlinked, they would become more useful—not only would recalling one fact prompt another but they would be less likely to be forgotten. This attempt to understand what is being learned is called '**deep learning**'.

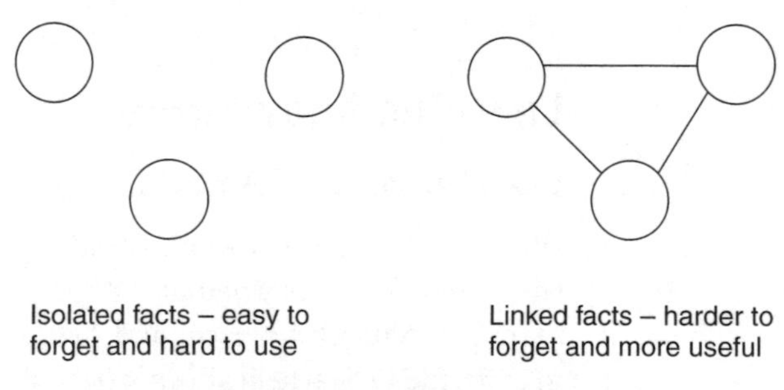

'Surface learning' vs 'deep learning'

If he had learned the lists and then tried out some simple clinical questions using the knowledge he had he might have found it easier to use it in the clinical setting. Finally, the knowledge that he learned was not incorporated in a very logical way. He now knows that hyperthyroidism is one of the causes of AF. However this knowledge may not link in with the information that he has stored away on hyperthyroidism. As a result when he sees a patient in the thyroid clinic with an irregular pulse, he won't consider AF.

The way in which our student links facts together affects how he retrieves them. If he has made some linkages that are wrong or has not made linkages he may end up thinking that ALL patients with AF should be anti-coagulated regardless. Not only will this stop him getting the right information out, it may mean that he gets the wrong information. As a student the worst that can happen is failing an exam or being made to feel foolish on a ward round (although that is bad enough). As a doctor the results can be extremely serious. Ensuring that our students understand information, see it in a clinical context, and apply it to problems is a key role for teachers.

A useful analogy for students is to compare medical knowledge to a town. It needs firm foundations, related services need to be close together, and you need to be able to get around easily. By building on what they already know, working to link knowledge together and applying what they have learned to clinical problems, students will be able to maximize the use of their time.

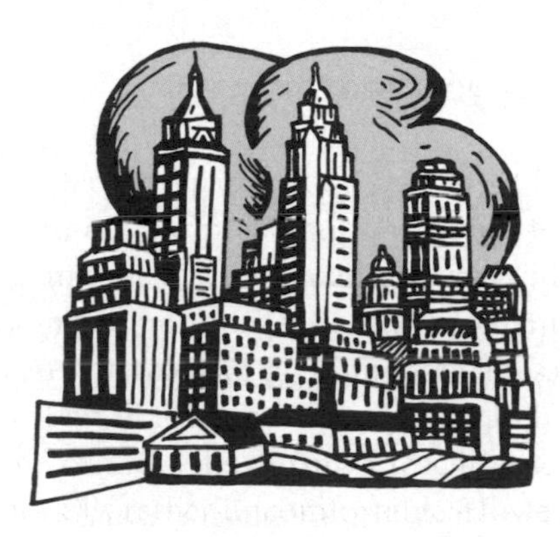

Medical knowledge is like a town: it needs firm foundations, related services close together, and excellent transport.

Teaching knowledge

How can we help students learn key facts as easily as possible and help them to use the information they have learned?

We know that in order to retain new knowledge students need to recall knowledge they already have, integrate the new information in a logical way, and then interact with it. Using the knowledge they have gained to solve problems will help them to apply it in the clinical setting. Remember that short-term memory is limited to seven chunks of information, and use this as a guide to the amount you can cover in a teaching segment.

The most efficient type of retrieval is recall, in which the information is found without any hints at all. Next is recognition, which means that when presented with the correct information among other pieces of information, the student recognizes the correct information. This is the type of retrieval commonly used in MCQ examinations. Sometimes knowledge can only be retrieved in the context in which it was learned. Other forms of retrieval are even less efficient and include reconstruction (where the information is slowly pieced together) and relearning. This latter is quicker than the initial learning but still slow.

Recall can be enhanced by repetition of information and subsequent rehearsal of information by the student. Information from the beginning and end of a session are best recalled, as is that which is important or interesting to the student. The more students are able to interact with the knowledge (by solving problems, self-testing) the better it will be recalled. Recall is reduced by inattention and poor concentration, and affected by the attitudes and emotions of the student during the initial session (Cotton, 1995).

As clinicians we know that it is not enough to know the facts, to be a good doctor you have to be able to use them. We call the understanding and application of knowledge '**higher level knowledge**'. Moving students beyond the simple memorization of facts is an important part of the teacher's role, discussed in Chapter 4 on basic teaching skills. Imparting information is relatively easy, although doing so in a way designed to maximize recall is more difficult. Harder still is encouraging students to understand new knowledge and go on to apply it. Asking probing questions stimulates students to interact with their knowledge and restructure it if necessary. Setting problems (particularly clinical cases) encourages students to use the information, and by putting it in context, may help recall in the clinical setting.

Structuring your teaching

You can enhance students' learning, subsequent recall, and application of knowledge by structuring your teaching in specific ways (see Chapter 3).

- Use an advance organizer. As new learning is built onto previous learning, it helps to alert students to what will be learned and allows them to call up any prior knowledge that may be relevant.
- Present information logically: this assists efficient retrieval.
- Highlight important information, and ensure the students understand why it is important. This will increase concentration and important facts are more likely to be recalled accurately.
- Site key information at the beginning and end of the session, ideally repeating it in the summary when closing the session.
- Allow students to interact with the knowledge by questioning/discussion/problem solving. This encourages them to move beyond simple recall of facts.
- Encourage the students to rehearse the knowledge and test themselves.

You can help students link knowledge together by making them interact with it. This is often done by the use of questions, prompting students towards solving a problem. While questioning, continually probe at the students understanding of a fact. It is very important to make sure that students don't have any serious misconceptions that will prevent them from correctly using knowledge, or from building onto what they already have. We are all familiar with giving students feedback on their examination skills, enabling them to perform the skill correctly in the future. Giving feedback on the underlying structure of students knowledge is just as vital, but often neglected.

Approaches to teaching knowledge

Teaching knowledge may range from telling students about the side-effects of digoxin during a ward round to organizing and teaching the pathology course. When considering how to teach a larger body of knowledge, two general approaches are used. Teachers can either give students a general overview of the field first and then fill in the details (general → specific), or they can give students a specific problem, and then fill in the knowledge around this, finally giving the overview (specific → general). This is shown below.

General → specific **Inductive reasoning**	**Specific → general** **Deductive reasoning**
Establish relevance.	Start with a practical problem.
Overview of area.	Look at areas of knowledge needed to explain problem.
Proceed in logical fashion (avoid too much detail initially).	'Put the jigsaw together' with knowledge overview.
Check for understanding.	Check for understanding.

There are merits to both approaches. One way to synthesize the two is to consider the amount of ground that students have to cover. In some cases, starting from the problem is rather like setting off on a journey without a map. If the potential content area is very large, the students may 'get lost' and explore only one corner of the area in detail, without realizing that there is still a long way to go. To avoid this you might want to use the general → specific approach at the start of a course. With this, you can map out what the students have to cover, and give them some idea of the depth to which they will be expected to go. In addition, if they have an overview of the content, they may be able to see possible links between pieces of knowledge that they might otherwise not relate together. Once they have a 'map' of the course, it may be better to switch to the specific → general approach, ensuring that the knowledge is grounded in context, and encouraging the students to start applying it immediately.

Commonly used techniques

The lecture

The traditional lecture is still widely used to disseminate knowledge. Giving a good lecture requires a lot of careful planning and preparation, and good presentation skills (see Chapter 6). To maximize learning find out exactly what the students have covered before and what the next speaker will do. This will ensure that you start off at the right level. It is helpful to give an advance organizer, as this will prime the student to start to learn. Unless you are giving the first lecture on a course, it makes sense to consider the specific → general approach. By starting off with a sample clinical case you make sure the students understand the clinical relevance of the information, and motivate them to listen to what you are saying. Consider providing lecture notes so the students can concentrate on what you are saying rather than writing, and complement your talk with clearly designed visual aids. As students cannot hold too much information in their short-term memory at once, break up your lecture into shorter chunks. Provide a short summary at the end of each chunk before continuing, and encourage application of knowledge rather than simple retention by some problem solving exercises. If presented in the form of a quiz, these will increase motivation. Finally, vary your teaching techniques to maintain the attention of students with different learning styles.

Maximizing learning in a lecture

- Advance organizer.
- Break information into chunks.
- Provide problem solving exercises.
- Use a variety of teaching styles.
- Reinforce with AV aids.
- Provide lecture notes.

Tutorials and seminars

Used in the right way, tutorials and seminars are an efficient way to encourage students to interact with information. To maximize learning in this setting, you might want to try a more student centred approach to teaching. Get students to set their own objectives. This is motivating and requires them to closely examine the knowledge they already have. You could move to a problem orientated approach (see below), or get students to read around the topic beforehand. This will oblige them to interact with the information more than they would in a lecture format. You can increase the challenge of sessions by assessing prior knowledge in detail and adjusting pitch, pace, and teaching style to the needs of the group. Lastly, you can probe students' understanding with questions, to ensure they fully understand the information.

Some tutorials are too long. You may want to pause in the middle, to keep you and your students comfortable, and prolong their effective learning time. Learning does not stop at the end of a tutorial, but goes on as students start to use their new information. Encourage them to use it as soon as possible—either by seeing patients, problem solving, or further reading.

Case presentations and conferences

Once more these terms are used interchangeably, but the technique used will be familiar to everyone. In most cases the student(s) present a case, which is then discussed by the facilitator and other students present. Properly managed case presentations are good for learning because they simulate 'real' medical practice, and thus your students will be able to recall the information easily in similar situations. Case presentations need careful stage-managing to make the most of their potential for learning—it is common for students to get interrupted and lose track of what they were saying, and for their hard work to be dismissed with a vague 'Well done'. Other students can be helped to learn from the case by using it to trigger a discussion and develop learning objectives for the group as a whole.

Maximizing learning in case presentations (Weinholtz and Edwards, 1992)

- Limit interruptions of the case presentation until the students have finished.
- Clarify any uncertainties about the case or terminology by questions from teacher and students.
- Use probing questions to ensure that the students understand the implications of the case.

- Use a white board or OHP to summarize key features of case and topic under discussion.
- Develop a series of objectives that the students 'need to know more about', and prioritize them.
- Give a short relevant talk on one or all of the objectives identified.
- Encourage the students to go away and read about the other areas identified.

Problem-based learning

Problem-based learning (PBL) has been around for over a decade in the UK, and is now used in many medical schools. This means that while students are often familiar with it, many teachers will not have come across it before. Your school may teach its entire curriculum through PBL, while others offer it only in some courses. Rather like seminars, PBL means different things in different places, but the key principles are that it is highly student centred, and that the learning derives from an initial problem (usually a clinical case).

Typical PBL would consist of the following stages (Bouhuijs *et al.*, 1987):

(1) Students read the case.

(2) Terms and concepts are clarified—students pick out words that are not understood and see if any group members can explain them.

(3) The case is discussed to define the problem.

(4) The case is analysed—possible explanations for the case are advanced.

(5) The possible explanations are collated (usually on a white board/flip chart) and linked together.

(6) Areas of uncertainty are defined and framed as clear questions or learning objectives.

(7) Students collect information on learning objectives.

(8) Information is synthesized and tested. The students report back and discuss new information to ensure that the case is now understood (it may be necessary to develop new learning objectives and find out further information at this stage).

PBL seems to help students learn because it is motivating, clinically orientated, and challenging. The motivation comes from the small group work, discussion, and effort of doing research, while the clinical scenarios make the work relevant. Because PBL requires students to set their own objectives they have to review their prior knowledge, and this not only primes them to learn but also means that the objectives are at an appropriate level. PBL also has advantages beyond the learning of knowledge. It improves communication skills, team-working, and equips students with the critical thinking and research skills they will need as life-long learners.

The exact definition (Maudsley, 1999a) and the theoretical basis for PBL have been hotly debated (Albanese, 2000), and while the most commonly cited theory is that of contextual learning (Coles, 1998) this has been criticized (Colliver, 2000) on the grounds of the poor research underlying contextual learning theory, and the contextualized nature of most medical learning. Other theoretical supports come from constructivism, information-processing theory

(Schmidt, 1983), co-operative learning, self-determination theory, and control theory. Of these, the first two provide support for the steps within PBL, while the second two explain the increased motivation which can be seen in PBL students.

The benefits and disadvantages of PBL have been discussed in depth and there are a series of reviews and meta-analyses which address the problem (Albanese and Mitchell, 1993; Vernon and Blake, 1993; Berkson, 1993; Norman and Schmidt, 1992). PBL seems to promote deep learning approach and the retention of knowledge. It is enjoyable and enhances the educational environment for students and staff. On the negative side, there are concerns about inadequate coverage of the syllabus and evidence that students from PBL courses find it stressful and can feel disadvantaged when compared with their colleagues (Woodward and Ferrier, 1983), although there is little evidence of a knowledge deficit. Ensuring coverage of the syllabus needs careful selection of problems, and student guidance about the relevant learning objectives. It is possible that the organization of information by students on PBL courses (the cognitive scaffolding) may be inadequate, and that this may inhibit further learning although research evidence is currently lacking. However, although students on PBL courses have done slightly better in some assessments (Blake *et al.*, 2000), there is no overwhelming evidence that PBL is superior to traditional educational methods in knowledge acquisition or clinical skills. Finally there are concerns about cost. It is likely that PBL programmes are more expensive in staff time, particularly for larger schools, although this has been debated (Nieuwenhuijzen Kruseman *et al.*, 1997). Uninterrupted face to face student teaching time is increased for each member of faculty involved, (Albanese and Mitchell, 1993) and there is more demand on library and computing facilities.

Being a PBL tutor

From the description of PBL above you can see that the tutor's role is not about imparting information, but about facilitating the group's learning. This can be frustrating, especially if the group seems to be spending a long time finding information that you know already. Students who are unfamiliar with PBL often find this frustrating too and often complain. It is important that they understand why they are doing PBL, and the first introductory session needs to be carefully handled.

Key areas to cover in the first PBL session

1. Introductions—spend time on this, especially if the group will be together for a whole course or year.
2. Ground rules of the group (punctuality, no interruptions, confidentiality, equal contributions to discussion, commitment to researching objectives identified by the group).
3. Ensure no timetabling clashes and check dates are correct.
4. What PBL is—a clear description of the process.
5. What is expected of the students.
6. What they can expect to gain from PBL.
7. How they will be assessed.
8. Ensure the written materials are understood by all.
9. Start the PBL process.

Once you have started your group off, it is tempting to imagine that you can just sit back and let the group continue. However, the tutors role in PBL is like a jigsaw with three key parts:

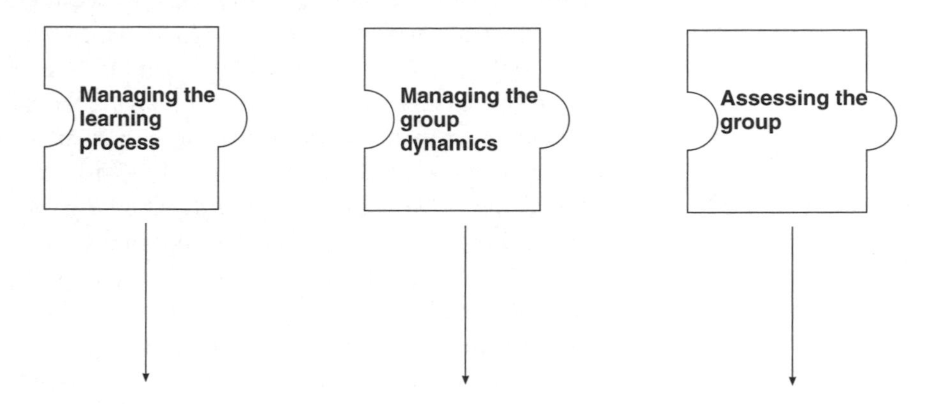

• Keep the learning moving (time and difficulty).	• Establish ground rules.	• Monitor individual progress.
• Ask probing questions to keep the students thinking at higher levels of knowledge.	• Ensure that tasks are fairly distributed—some will be harder than others.	• Get students to reflect on how they solved the problem and consider improvements.
• Encourage students to summarize periodically.	• Create a 'safe' learning environment.	• Give constructive feedback on performance.
• Make sure students can access learning resources.	• Involve all students in discussion.	• Complete formal assessments.
• Keep presentations short and relevant.	• Assist student 'leaders' and 'scribes'.	
• Make sure information is correct.	• Use your facilitation skills.	

This is a daunting list, and novice tutors often say 'It would be quicker just to tell them' or 'What am I there for?' It is certainly true that tutors in PBL groups spend less time talking than they would in a lecture, but that does not mean that the students are learning less.

PBL is not one form of teaching but occupies a spectrum from the tutor centred to the student centred. In the more tutor centred types, you will be the person leading the debate and probably summarizing the discussion on the white board. Often as a novice tutor this feels more comfortable as you still 'feel like a teacher'. In student centred PBL the students will elect their own leader and scribe, and your role will be to monitor the groups progress. However you still have a key role guiding the group, and keeping them on the right track. A lot of the benefits of PBL are lost if the group does not function well, or if it goes off on the wrong track due to misconceptions. You need to pay close attention to spot when and why a group is going off track, and use questions with care to bring them back.

You will feel more confident if the case is in your area of expertise, and in this case you could call yourself a '**content expert**' or '**expert tutor**'. However many schools have used non-expert tutors with great success. While it can be very daunting to facilitate a case about which you know little, you should have good tutor's notes to help you, and it is a great opportunity to learn.

Corrective feedback from tutors is key to PBL. Without feedback, groups may fail to solve problems or develop incorrect conceptual or procedural understandings. This may prevent them from solving future problems (Needham and Begg, 1991). This has led to great debate about the use of expert versus non-expert tutors (Maudsley, 1999b). Using non-expert tutors is very attractive for a medical school as it offers greater flexibility in scheduling. It also offers groups the advantage of having the same tutor over time. The different tutors seem to have effects in the two areas of facilitation and eventual content knowledge. Expert tutors tend to be more directive (Silver and Wilkerson, 1993), and their groups generate more learning issues (Eagle *et al.*, 1992). Despite this they are rated more highly by students. Most studies have found that students taught by experts have equivalent or better knowledge than students taught by non-experts, particularly where students prior knowledge is poor or the course poorly structured (Schmidt *et al.*, 1993). Some schools have experimented with tutorless PBL, but the evidence about its effectiveness is unclear (Neville, 1999). It is likely that novice students are more in need of tutors who are able to be structured and directive. As the students acquire more knowledge, both in medicine and about the PBL process, they probably have less need of an expert tutor.

Writing a problem

In many schools a bank of problems already exists. These will be continuously updated following student feedback, and you may be asked to contribute. It is a good idea to get a small and multidisciplinary group of teaching colleagues together, as you will be able to share resources and ideas. We would suggest the following steps:

- Check what objectives you are required to cover (these may not exist and you will then have to develop them yourselves).
- Check what form of assessment the students will be facing—this may influence the type of problem you use.
- Devise possible cases by discussion in your group—the cases need to be interesting and sufficiently complex for the level of student.
- Select the most promising case and write a succinct summary.
- Try it out on other colleagues/medical students to see if they can identify the learning objectives you wanted.
- Identify the resources required, and check when resource people are contactable.
- Write the student materials and a tutors guide.
- Ensure that the new question is included in the course evaluation.

A tutors guide should contain a brief overview of what PBL is and administrative information about timetabling and the group members. It should have the initial case, aims, detailed objectives, and useful prompt questions that novice tutors can use if the students seem very stuck. It may contain supplementary information that the tutor can reveal after certain initial discussions have taken place. Finally, it should have a list of resources and some background information for tutors. This is particularly useful if you are using non-expert tutors.

A sample PBL problem and learning objectives are shown below.

Initial problem

You are a GP. At the end of a busy surgery you see Yasmin, who is 14 years old. She tells you that she wants to go on the pill because she is having sex with her boyfriend and does not want to get pregnant. She is insistent that her parents must not know. She seems sensible and reasonably well informed. What do you do?

Supplementary information

On questioning Yasmin tells you that her period is about two weeks late.

Learning objectives

1 To understand the pros and cons of different modes of contraception.
2 To understand the mode of action of oral contraception.
3 To understand indications and contraindications of oral contraception.
4 To understand consent in children.
5 To understand the duty of confidentiality towards children.
6 To explore the issues of teenage pregnancy and abortion.

Additional information for tutors might include more detailed learning objectives: for example 'To outline the principle requirements in UK law for informed consent in underage children with specific reference to Gillick competency'. It could also include sample prompt questions: for example 'Can you give Yasmin the pill without telling her parents?'

If your school is developing a PBL course then it is vital to ensure content validity using a 'blueprinting' approach (see Chapter 9, p. 152). Starting PBL from scratch takes a lot of time in both question development and staff development.

Computer-assisted learning

Computers are now ubiquitous, and many students may have their own. Your medical school will have several well equipped computer laboratories and most students are familiar with email, the Internet, Medline, word-processing and data-handling programmes. Many medical schools have developed and use computer-assisted learning packages. These vary in quality, but have great potential for learning.

The best CAL programmes are clinically based, supplement well written text with good quality photos or video, and are interactive. They adjust the level of the programme to the ability of the user by monitoring their answers to questions. This maintains the level of challenge without leaving the learner behind. Their flexibility means that students can use them when they like and at their own pace. Relevance is assured by their clinical focus and many of them offer the student the chance to make mistakes in safety and see what the consequences would be. As the quality of programmes improves they will be increasingly used, particularly as they can be adapted to keep up with medical developments at little additional cost. The drawback of CAL is that it does not develop skills or many of the necessary generic competencies that practicing doctors need.

As a medical teacher you can help students by testing programmes first to see whether they are appropriate, and then guiding students to the best programmes for them. It may be useful for students to read around a topic before they start or supplement a programme with clinical experience (for example a visit to an appropriate outpatient clinic). Writing a CAL programme is covered in Chapter 6 on audio-visual aids.

Independent study

Much learning in medical schools is done outside of formal lectures and small group sessions. This is increasingly recognized and protected time is allocated for private study during the day (Dent and Harden, 2001). Students may be triggered to learn by a forthcoming exam, by an interesting case on the ward, to keep up with their friends, or by a charismatic teacher. We usually notice this learning only when it doesn't happen—when a student fails examinations, or develops psychological problems. You may be asked to talk to a student who has had difficulties and you will find that they have problems in one or more of the following areas (Newble and Cannon, 1994):

(a) Social factors: too much time spent on social activities, family or money problems, poor accommodation.

(b) Psychological factors: undue anxiety, personal problems, depression.

(c) Specific study skills problems: lack of study plan, inappropriate environment, poor time management, difficulties in setting and prioritizing objectives, use of inappropriate resources, poor examination technique.

There may be little that you can do about students' social and psychological problems, but your medical school will have student support and counselling services available. Many students who have previously coped well with their studies develop problems at medical school. They often feel overwhelmed by the amount of information they are expected to retain, and abandon deep learning strategies for surface ones. While this will get them through the next exam, they then find it harder to use the information later on. Developing good study habits is very important for medical students. They need to be able to work effectively and efficiently. Many medical schools include sessions on study skills in their introductory courses.

Independent study is often seen as a time when students 'get on with it'. However there is a lot that teachers can do to help students learn effectively. Recognizing the role of independent learning and timetabling it into the day is vital. However there is no use in doing this if the students do not have access to somewhere they can work. Make sure that the library is open at the times you have scheduled. Lastly, make sure that your students have got the study skills that they need, either from an initial study skills course, from leaflets, or by refreshing their memories with a special session.

Learning skills

Types of skills

Doctors have a lot of skills to learn. When medical students think about medical skills they usually include:

- History taking.
- Physical examination.
- Diagnostic and therapeutic skills.
- Resuscitation skills.

However there are other essential clinical skills which are sometimes called '**generic competencies**'. They include:

- Communication skills.
- Critical thinking and problem solving.

- Team-working, organization, and management.
- Information technology.
- Professional attitudes and awareness of the ethical basis of health care.

When we think about teaching skills it is important to include generic competencies as well as clinical skills

Learning a basic skill

In its simplest form a skill is a pattern of movements that when put together achieve an aim. For example, a child learns that the following sequence of pencil strokes, when put together in the right order, make the capital letter A.

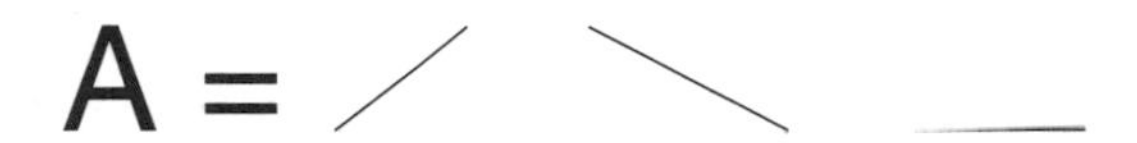

A child can learn to write his or her name well before they can read or write anything else by memorizing the sequence of strokes. However for this skill to be useful in communication a child has to learn further skills: to associate the letters with their sounds, to be able to decipher phonemes, and to read. Once this has been achieved the child can start to write down their own thoughts and ideas like:

riting is difficut

This shows that the skill of writing has been acquired but some knowledge about the peculiarities of English spelling and grammar is needed. Eventually the child is able to write:

Writing is difficult.

Being able to write, like most skills, needs a synthesis of psychomotor skills and knowledge. Once we have mastered the skill and use it regularly we become '**experts**'. As experts we perform the skill unconsciously, automatically adjusting for unexpected changes. Learners or '**novices**' have to think carefully about what they are doing, and if something unexpected happens, they may have to start from scratch again. Because experts do the skill unconsciously, they may find it difficult to break the skill down into its component parts.

Learning complex skills

If writing is difficult, how much more difficult are the tasks we require medical students and doctors to perform. While many studies look at 'pure' skills (i.e. the psychomotor part of the skill), in reality we perform highly integrated skills guided by our knowledge. The more complex the skill, the harder it is to learn. As a result the most difficult skill for a medical student to learn is the medical interview, as this requires the integration of communication skills, medical knowledge, problem solving, and physical examination.

Some of factors that help students to learn knowledge are also true of skills. It is often helpful for a student to be able to relate the new skill to something that they are already familiar with. For example, when learning to suture, it may be helpful to check whether the student can sew: there are similarities in the skills which can be highlighted and make a useful starting point. If a skill is simple a student can be expected to learn it all in one go. However with more complex skills, it makes sense to break them up into chunks. A student who wants to perform a caesarean needs some basic skills (like suturing) first.

Just as it is easier to learn facts if they are presented logically, so it is easier to learn a skill if the student is shown the skill clearly. While it is possible (although not advisable) to learn medical knowledge entirely from books, learning a physical skill requires hands-on experience. Just practise alone is not enough however. Without feedback, a student may be able to approximate what you are doing, but not well enough to competently perform the skill. Once a skill has been learned and reinforced by practise it is difficult to change (as any musician or golfer will know). It is far better to get it right first time, and feedback in the early stages of learning a skill is vital.

To make sure that the skill is retained a students needs to practise and to keep on practising. You may not have forgotten how to ride your bike, but you will probably have a test-run before you embark on a 50 mile charity ride. The same is true of medical skills, especially those that might be needed in an emergency. This is why resuscitation certificates need regular renewing.

Traditionally medical skills teaching relied on the 'see one, do one, teach one' principle, which is no longer ethically or medico-legally defensible. Considerable work has been done on the theory of skills acquisition and teaching (Patrick, 1992), with the emphasis recently on the intellectual and cognitive aspects of more complex tasks. It is likely that skills learning also occurs by the development of schemata that are fine tuned until the task becomes automatic. It is the teachers task to ensure that the correct schemata develop, that they are linked together appropriately, and that the student understands when he has reached a level at which he can function independently.

Several models of teaching are useful in skills acquisition (Patrick, 1992) but the most frequently encountered is Peyton's four stage approach (Peyton, 1998), which is widely used in Advanced Life Support Training (leading to it often being called the ATLS model). This involves demonstrations, first without and then with explanations, followed by a demonstration where the learner describes each step, and finally guided 'hands-on' experience. The first demonstration provides the learner with an overview of the skill performed normally, while the slower second demonstration permits the student a clearer idea of the cognitive processes underlying the manoeuvres. The third step allows the student to start interacting with the new information they have just acquired, while the fourth stage moves the student on to integrating the necessary cognitive and psychomotor skills. Immediate application of the new skill is important in retention, and repetitive practise (overtraining) (Patrick, 1992) in different situations reinforces the skill and speeds the acquisition of expertise.

In a complex task, task analysis (a learning hierarchy analysis applied to a skill) is used to enumerate all the steps of a procedure. Procedural-prerequisite relations describe the links between the steps (i.e. you must do X before Y), whereas procedural-decision relations describe changes to the procedure made in different settings (i.e. if you find A you had better do X rather than Z) (Dent and Harden, 2001). An alternative method, the simple-to-complex model (Reigeluth, 1999), starts with the simplest practical application of the task and then increases the complexity and diversity of the task until the learner is fully competent.

Teaching skills

Because there are similarities between learning knowledge and learning skills, some of the approaches described above are also used. In the setting of a skills laboratory, or with a co-operative patient in protected time it is possible to teach a skill very comprehensively using the following process.

1 Activation of prior knowledge.

2 Silent demonstration.

3 Demonstration with commentary.

4 Demonstration with student commentary.

5 Supervised practise by student.

Activating prior knowledge is not only useful to fit the new skill into the right area of memory, but it will also help the student relate the new task to something they can do already.

Activating prior knowledge in ophthalmoscopy

Cognitive domain

Question: When have you seen doctors using ophthalmoscopes?
What were they looking for?

Skills domain

Question: Have you ever looked through a keyhole?
How close to the keyhole do you need to get to see the room beyond?

For the student to be able to perform the whole task they need to know what it looks like. Even if the task is long, they will need at some point to have an overview of what they are aiming towards. If the task is very long and complex it is a good idea for you to break it up into chunks. This is easier if you write out a list of all the things that the students must do and then divide it logically. You must ensure that the student can 'weld' these chunks back together again. If time allows it is a good idea for the first demonstration to be 'silent': that is to say you carry on as if the student is not there.

You should then do a second demonstration where you talk about what you are doing. This is very important, not only because it is not always easy to see what a demonstrator is doing but also because it explains and reinforces what is going on—the student is getting input both visually and aurally.

A third demonstration should then be done with the student describing what the teacher is doing. This helps the student remember the different steps, and what they are for. Finally, the student can 'have a go'. It is tempting to leave at this point, but in fact the most important part of the teaching process is the feedback to students on what they are doing and how to improve their performance. Without this they can get into bad habits that will interfere with their performance and will be difficult to unlearn at a later stage. Feedback during skills training should follow the general rules of feedback, but try and save your feedback until the student has finished. If you continuously feedback during the performance, it inhibits learning the skill.

If you have been teaching venesection in the skills laboratory and you are confident that your students are now competent, it is important that they now have the chance to practise their skills in the clinical setting. Ideally they want to do this in the next few days, while the skills and confidence they have acquired are still fresh. Spending the morning with the phlebotomist and the afternoon helping the SHO in casualty will provide initial experience, but they need to practise the skills until they are expert and then maintain them. If a student will need to use a skill in several scenarios, they should be encouraged to practise it in each one as far as possible. After each performance of the skill encourage them to reflect on what more they have learned.

Teaching skills in the clinical setting

In many situations you will not have time to go through the full demonstration/practise process: you may be on a ward round or in morning surgery. How can you maximize skill acquisition in this setting? Often you won't have to go through the whole process; the students are no longer complete novices, but have a little skill and want to develop it. We have found that the following approach is helpful:

1. Let the student set the agenda: 'I want you to think about what was most difficult for you, and we will focus on that'.
2. Get the student to demonstrate the skill while talking you through what they are doing.
3. Closely observe the student performing.
4. Give constructive feedback.
5. Let the student try again with more feedback.
6. Encourage him to practise after the session and learn some more about the skill (if appropriate).

Teaching communication skills and the medical interview

Until recently, consultation and communication skills were not differentiated. Consultation skills are what we do in the medical interview (take a history, discuss management), while communication skills describe what we do when we interact with people (patients, relatives, and colleagues) generally. As clinicians we know that good communication is the cornerstone of medical practice. Unfortunately you will come across students who see communication skills training as an unnecessary extra within the curriculum. Teaching a difficult subject may be made harder by students who are not motivated to learn.

The medical interview

There are many models of consultation skills available to students (Pendleton *et al.*, 1984; Neighbour, 1992; Stewart *et al.*, 1995). Your medical school will have embraced one of them, and it is important that you are familiar with the terminology you are expected to use. All of them emphasize the importance of seeing the patient as a person, understanding their ideas and concerns about the problem, and their expectations about what can be done. They stress the importance of helping the patient to an understanding of their complaint, and negotiating a management plan.

A consultation has some basic tasks. These are (Kurtz *et al.*, 1998):

- Initiating the session.
- Gathering information.
- Building the relationship.
- Explanation and planning.
- Closing the session.

For both students and teachers having a clear structure for complex task is very important. Consultations can be affected by their content and emotions that arise. Once the basic skills have been mastered, students can go on to deal with more complex skills such as breaking bad news and dealing with angry patients.

Teaching communication skills

The basics of communication skills (verbal and non-verbal communication) may be taught in isolation, but most medical schools move students quickly on to putting their knowledge into practice. As with all skills learning students need to understand what they are trying to achieve, and practise the skill with feedback. Unfortunately a consultation is so complex that it is difficult for students to 'see' what they are doing, and an observer who can give high quality feedback is essential. Medical schools have revolutionized consultation and communication skills teaching by the use of role play, simulated patients, and video in the communication skills laboratory (see Chapter 8). The advantages of role play and simulated patients are that students can make mistakes in safety and are able to 'replay' situations until they are comfortable.

Teaching in the clinical setting has the advantage of using real patients. This raises the challenge for students, but requires close surveillance by staff to ensure that the patients are comfortable. You will have limits on your time and so the pragmatic approach used by most teachers is to 'chunk' the consultation. This means to cut the consultation into smaller parts—'Spend 5 minutes asking Mr. X about his chest pain'. Many teachers then use this as a springboard to explore knowledge domains related to the subject. Using some of the time to feedback on the student's observed consultation skills will make the most of their experience.

Teaching communication skills on the ward

Show that you value communication skills.

Try and model good communication skills for the students.

Get students to take 'chunks' of the history.

Feedback on communication skills, including the patient's input if appropriate.

Look at key features of the history and discuss how best to explore them.

Consider short role plays explaining diagnosis/management to the patient.

Teaching clinical reasoning

Once clinicians have gathered information from the patient, they use this to reach a working diagnosis, to decide whether to start therapy or whether to admit a patient. Experienced clinicians seem to use two main methods to arrive at a diagnosis—pattern recognition in easy cases and the generation and testing of hypotheses in difficult cases (Elstein and Schwaz, 2002). For students all cases are difficult—they haven't seen enough clinical material to use pattern recognition.

This process of generating and testing hypotheses (the hypothetico deductive model) is difficult for students to learn, and this seems to stem from the fact that students and clinicians acquire and process information from their patients in different ways.

Experienced clinicians	Students
• Take patient information.	• Take a history as a list of pre-set questions one by one.
• Reflect on it during the consultation.	• Examine the patient completely as a pre-set series of steps.
• Plan new questions during the consultation.	• Reflect on the information gleaned after the consultation.
• Test out their hypothesis during the consultation.	• Come up with a hypothesis after the consultation.
	• Cannot test the hypothesis with further questions unless they return to the patient.
	• Gather so much data they cannot see the wood for the trees.

There is no doubt that students adopt this method of data collection because we teach them to take histories and examine in this way. We then reward them for presenting cases in exhaustive detail. To improve their clinical reasoning skills we need to get students to gather information in a different way.

Practicing clinicians are faster than students at reaching a diagnosis, even in a difficult case, because they start making differential diagnoses almost immediately (Elstein *et al.*, 1978). They can do this because within the first few moments of a medical interview they identify the 'diagnostic ball park' the patient is in, and tailor their questions appropriately. This ball park is a formulation of the presenting complaint such as 'This is about chronic diarrhoea'.

To improve students' clinical reasoning, it helps to get them into the right diagnostic ball park as early as possible. It is easiest to do this when you are observing them interviewing a patient. Get them to focus on the key features of each presenting complaint before they start to ask questions. The key features of each presenting complaint are contained within the mnemonic SSSTOP.

S	Symptoms	The characteristics of the symptoms. Associated symptoms.
S	Severity	
S	Situational factors	Precipitating factors. Exacerbating factors. Relieving factors.
T	Time course	Duration. Constant or intermittent. Previous episodes or not.
O	Onset	Sudden. Gradual.
P	Patient characteristics	Demographics—age, race, sex. Risk behaviours.

Once students have identified the ball park they can start making hypotheses. These may be few and illogical—'It could be Crohns disease, an infection, or a tumour' but show that they are starting to generate hypotheses. By applying a rational method of hypothesis generation (the 'surgical sieve'—considering possibilities under the heading of infectious, metabolic, neoplastic, etc.) students may be able to generate more hypotheses to test. Encourage the students to summarize the presenting complaint into one sentence, and then encourage them to:

- **Reflect**—and consider what diagnoses come to mind when 'hearing' the early representation.
- **Plan**—what further questions or examination would help them establish a diagnoses.
- **Experiment**—proceed with further questions and examination, to test the hypothesis.

Once they have collected all the information they can, the student can start to use it to solve the problem. There are two basic reasoning approaches to diagnosis used in medicine: forward reasoning (data-driven hypothesis) and backward reasoning (hypothesis driven). In the first, the student looks at all the information and then concludes that the patient has diagnosis A. In backward reasoning the student looks at the patient and decides he could have diagnosis A because he has symptoms B and C. Experts use forward reasoning and we should encourage students to do the same. However, students often do not have enough knowledge to use forward reasoning, and may use backward reasoning. This technique may be quicker, but is more prone to error, as all the information is not taken into account. We should encourage students to use forward reasoning when they have enough information.

As with all skills, clinical reasoning improves with practice. Not only do students become quicker, but as they see more cases, they also start to develop an in-depth knowledge of the ways in which common illnesses present, allowing them to recognize problems very quickly. This technique is called 'pattern recognition'. Developing pattern recognition is speeded up if you expose students frequently to common problems, and gradually increase the complexity of each case. It also helps to teach students to recognize the discriminating features that enable them to distinguish between diagnoses, rather than trying to memorize the specific features of each diagnosis. Teaching clinical reasoning in practice is covered in more depth in Chapter 8, Teaching in the clinical setting.

Learning and teaching attitudes

Having the right attitudes is an important part of being a doctor, and these have been listed by the GMC (General Medical Council, 1998). The problem with attitudes is that they are invisible—only appearing in the way that they affect our behaviour. Not only that but they vary depending on the situation, and may be masked in research by people answering questions in 'socially acceptable' ways.

Students learn from many sources at medical school. Some of this learning is intended and planned (the curriculum) and the rest is often termed the '**hidden curriculum**'. There is no doubt that during medical school there is an increase in negative attitudes (e.g. cynicism). Students must learn these from somewhere, and as they are not part of the taught curriculum, they must come from other interactions with staff.

How do we ensure that doctors have the right attitudes (Martin *et al.*, 2002)? As attitudes are relatively fixed over time, perhaps one way would be to select students who already have the views required. Unfortunately we don't know exactly what attitudes we require, and we can't be sure that we can detect them accurately. If we cannot select for positive attitudes, we need to teach them. As a lot of the current undesirable learning stems from the hidden curriculum, a medical school needs staff that are able to model desirable attitudes, both to patients and to their students (e.g. by not humiliating them). This needs staff development and committed leadership.

In order to learn we need to interact with information. By not discussing attitudes and ethical dilemmas we risk our students not modifying their attitudes at all. Because attitudes are highly personal, discussion is only likely to take place in the (very) small group setting, and when the student feels safe. During the discussion a student can reveal his attitudes and monitor the responses of others to them. Role play is useful as it allows students to experience another's situation. Discussion with a mentor may help students address their attitudinal and ethical dilemmas.

Some schools have developed specific courses (particularly on ethics), although if not compulsory and not assessed these can suffer from poor attendance. Other schools rely on the attitude teaching inherent in some courses (for example consultation skills teaching).

Teaching attitudes

1 Ensure that you comply with the requirements of 'Good Medical Practice'.
2 Treat students with respect and consideration.
3 Offer students time to discuss ethical dilemmas as they arise.
4 Encourage students to attend medical ethics courses.
5 Ensure that students medico-legal knowledge base (confidentiality, consent, etc.) is adequate.

Conclusion

The content of a session influences the teaching strategies you will use to help students learn. Interaction with information, whether knowledge, skills, or attitudes is what brings about change, and structuring your teaching to maximize this interaction will help your students learn.

Practical tips for maximizing learning

1 Activate prior knowledge.
2 Present new information in small chunks.
3 Allow the students time to integrate new skills/information.
4 Encourage the students to work with the new skills/information by applying it.
5 Feedback to students on their progress.
6 Encourage continued learning after the session ends.

References

Albanese, M. (2000) PBL: why curricula are likely to show little effect on knowledge and skills. *Med Educ* **34**, 729–38.

Albanese, M. A., and Mitchell, S. (1993) Problem-based learning: a review of literature on its outcomes and implementation issues. *Acad Med* **68**, 52–81.

Berkson, L. (1993) Problem based learning: have expectations been met? *Acad Med* **68**, S79–88.

Blake, R. L., Hosokawa, E. D., and Riley, S. (2000) Student performance on Step 1 and Step 2 of the United States Medical Licensing Examination following implementation of a problem-based learning curriculum. *Acad Med* **75**, 66–70.

Bouhuijs, P., Schmidt, H. G., and van Berkel, H. (1987) *Problem-based learning as an educational strategy*. Maastricht, Netherlands: Network Publications.

Coles, C. (1998) How medical students learn. In *Medical education in the millennium* (ed. B. Jolly and L. Rees), pp. 61–82. Oxford: Oxford University Press.

Colliver, J. A. (2000) The effectiveness of a problem-based learning curricula: research and theory. *Acad Med* **75**, 259–99.

Cotton, J. (1995) *The theory of learning: an introduction*. London: Kogan Page.

Dent, J. A., and Harden, R. (2001) *A practical guide for medical teachers*. Edinburgh: Churchill Livingstone.

Eagle, C. J., Harasym, P., and Mandin, H. (1992) Effects of tutors with case expertise on problem-based learning issues. *Acad Med* **67**, 465–9.

Elstein, A. S., and Schwaz, A. (2002) Clinical problem solving and diagnostic decision making: selective review of the cognitive literature. *Br Med J* **324**, 729–32.

Elstein, A. S., Shulman, L. S., and Sprafka, S. A. (1978) *Medical problem solving: an analysis of clinical reasoning*. Harvard, Mass.: Harvard University Press.

General Medical Council. (1998) *Good medical practice*. London: General Medical Practice.

Kurtz, S., Silverman, J., and Draper, J. (1998) *Teaching and learning communication skills in medicine*. Oxford: Radcliffe Medical Press.

Martin, J., Lloyd, M., and Singh, S. (2002) Professional attitudes: can they be taught and assessed in medical education. *Clin Med* **2**, 17–23.

Maudsley, G. (1999a) Do we all mean the same thing by 'problem-based learning'? A review of the concepts and a formulation of the ground rules. *Acad Med* **74**, 178–85.

Maudsley, G. (1999b) Roles and responsibilities of the problem based learning tutor in the undergraduate medical curriculum. *Br Med J* **318**, 657–61.

Needham, D., and Begg, I. (1991) Problem orientated training promotes spontaneous analogical transfer: memory orientated training promotes memory for training. *Mem Cognit* **19**, 543–57.

Neighbour, R. (1992) *The inner consultation*. London: Kluwer Academic.

Neville, A. J. (1999) The problem-based learning tutor: teacher? facilitator? evaluator? *Med Teach* **21**, 393–401.

Newble, D., and Cannon, R. (1994) *A handbook for medical teachers*, 3rd edn. London: Kluwer Academic Publishers.

Nieuwenhuijzen Kruseman, A. C., Kolle, L. F., and Scherpbier, A. (1997) Problem-based learning at Maastricht—an assessment of cost and outcome. *Educ Health* **10**, 179–87.

Norman, G. R., and Schmidt, H. G. (1992) The psychological basis of problem-based learning: a review of the evidence. *Acad Med* **67**, 557–65.

Patrick, J. (1992) *Training, research and practice.* London: Academic Press.

Pendleton, D., Schofield, T., Tate, P., and Havelock, P. (1984) *The consultation: an approach to teaching and learning.* Oxford: Oxford University Press.

Peyton, J. W. R. (1998) *Teaching and learning in medical practice.* Rickmansworth, Herts: Manticore Europe Limited.

Reigeluth, C. M. (1999) The elaboration theory. In *Instructional design theories and models volume 2: a new paradigm of instructional theory* (ed. C. M. Reigeluth), pp. 425–54. New Jersey: Lawrence Erlbaum Associates.

Schmidt, H. G. (1983) Problem-based learning: rationale and description. *Med Educ* **17**, 11–6.

Schmidt, H. G., van der Arend, A., Moust, J. H., Kokx, I., and Boon, L. (1993) Influence of tutor's subject matter expertise on students effort and achievement in problem-based learning. *Acad Med* **68**, 784–91.

Silver, M., and Wilkerson, L. A. (1993) Effects of tutors with subject expertise on the problem-based tutorial process. *Acad Med* **66**, 298–300.

Stewart, M., Brown, J. B., Weston, W. W., McWhinney, I. R., Mc William, C. L., and Freeman, T. R. (1995) *Patient-centred consultation: transforming the clinical method.* Thousand Oaks: Sage Publications Inc.

Vernon, D. T. A., and Blake, R. L. (1993) Does problem-based learning work? A meta-analysis of evaluative research. *Acad Med* **68**, 550–63.

Weinholtz, D., and Edwards, J. (1992) Teaching in the conference room. In *Teaching during rounds: a handbook for attending physicians and residents* (ed. D. Weinholtz and J. Edwards). Baltimore: The John Hopkins University Press.

Woodward, C. A., and Ferrier, B. M. (1983) The content of the medical curriculum at McMaster university: graduates' evaluation of their preparation for post-graduate training. *Med Educ* **17**, 54–60.

Acknowledgement

We are grateful for the input of Dr. Jonathan Martin MMedSci (Clin Ed), MRCGP, ILTM, Senior Teaching Fellow, Royal Free and University College Medical School, London, with the writing of this chapter.

CHAPTER 6

Designing and using teaching materials

'A picture is worth a thousand words.'

Having prepared and planned your session, you might think that with adequate teaching skills you can make a success of anything. However any teaching session, no matter how well delivered, will fall flat if the teaching materials that accompany it are poor. Making high quality teaching materials that help students learn is a skill that improves with practise. While some of you will have a gift for producing materials that are visually attractive, others will find that this is difficult. This eye for graphic design is very useful, but even if you have no abilities in that direction at all, this chapter will help you select the most appropriate teaching material for your session and design new materials.

Why use teaching materials?

From our understanding of cognitive processes in learning (see Chapter 2) we know that what is seen and heard becomes part of the internal processing of a student, facilitating the construction of meaning. Teaching materials can contribute to the learning process by providing the stimulus (Ausubel *et al.*, 1978) or explanation to trigger deep cognitive processing on the part of the learner therefore enabling the build up of a knowledge structure by both visual and auditory information (Rumelhart, 1980). Understanding how students learn puts us in a strong position to know how to design materials that enable us to teach more effectively in a way that improves communication and facilitates learning. Although teaching materials have the potential to contribute to learning, whether they do or not depends on the way they have been designed and are used.

Five trends have been identified in instructional material development that mirror some of the more general trends in medical education (Laidlaw, 1995). These move from:

low technology	→	high technology
fixed resource	→	flexible resource
subject expert	→	educational technologist
content related	→	study guide
creative approach	→	educational approach

Traditional written learning material in medical education has usually been very much towards the left side of the spectra. Moving to the right-hand side will produce materials designed to promote effective learning that are more engaging for the student.

Several educational models have been proposed to help material design. One of the simplest models is Laidlaw and Hardens' 'FAIR principles' (Laidlaw, 1995), derived from the work of Gagné (Gagné *et al.*, 1988), and particularly useful in the design of study guides and handouts. They emphasize the importance of:

providing **F**eedback
integrating **A**ctivity
Individualizing your material
ensuring **R**elevance in your materials

Producing materials that actively promote learning is more cost-effective than just producing factual material that could be found elsewhere.

Choosing teaching materials

As technology advances there are an increasing number of educational resources available to both tutors and students. The difficulty now faced by many tutors is how to choose the most appropriate teaching materials.

Before making your choice of teaching material it may be useful to ask yourself:

- What am I trying to achieve—is it to introduce variety, stimulate discussion, or reinforce ideas?
- Should I mix different materials to cater for different learning styles and preferences?
- Do any of my learning objectives for the session already dictate the use of a particular material?
- Do both the teacher and the students have the access and skills to use this medium?
- What is already available from colleagues/the Internet, etc.?
- What can I afford in both time invested and money?

It is tempting to develop complicated and expensive materials just because the technology is there to make it possible. This may not always be the best use of your resources, especially if the materials are so complex that the students find them hard to use.

It does not necessarily follow that high technology options are the best. Be sparing with modern technology as it is easy to get carried away by the medium and forget the message.

Audio-visual aids

Audio-visual aids have been part of the teaching process for many years. In years gone by teachers used blackboard and chalk. Technological advances mean there are more choices available, but it does not mean that they are always better. The basic principle to keep in mind is that audio-visual aids should be just that: audio or visual and they should aid—not hinder.

Chalk and talk—blackboards, white boards, and flip charts

Blackboards

The blackboard is one of the oldest audio-visual aids, using the combination of the teachers voice with writing on the board. It is still in use today and has stood the test of time for a number of reasons, probably the main one being that it is very cheap. With this method a major advantage is that the information can evolve and so can be used very effectively to encourage audience participation. As the information does not have to be predetermined, it is an excellent choice of material for brainstorming ideas and gathering information from participants in a group. Although it is common for the tutor to do the writing, this does not have to be the case and encouraging a student to write is one way of ensuring involvement.

The main disadvantage is the relative lack of permanence of the information. Writing must be mainly generated during the teaching session and as there is a limit to the space available at one time, layout and content must be considered if important messages are not to be lost from view.

The principles of white boards and flip charts are similar. White boards have little advantage over blackboards. In fact they have disadvantages—they require special pens that are liable to run out with little warning. You must also check that the pens you are intending to use are suitable for a white board and will not stain it permanently.

Flip charts

Flip charts are more versatile. They can provide almost unlimited space for writing which does not have to be deleted before more can be added. The information produced can all be viewed at once if completed sheets are placed around the walls and the information can also be retained (although in a rather cumbersome way) for use again at a later date. Sections of paper can be removed to aid small group work which can also be viewed by the whole group. Flip charts can also be moved around the classroom but be careful to ensure visibility. If you are right handed, you should place the board at the front to right side of a group and stand on the right in order to avoid obstructing the view as you write. The opposite is true for left handers. As with all of these methods legibility is essential, and clear writing in a colour that can be seen from the back of the room is required.

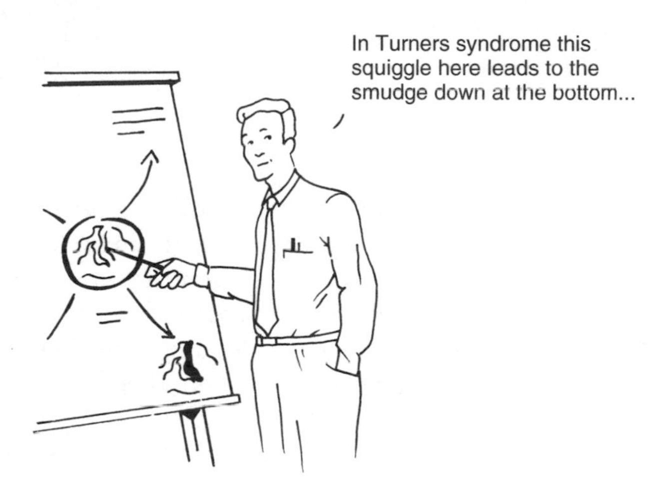

Overhead transparencies

The overhead projector is a popular and widely used teaching aid (Laidlaw, 1987a). It may appear old-fashioned and less impressive compared with more modern technology—but it is very effective and reliable. Most institutions have at least one projector. They are relatively cheap and require little maintenance. On the whole, overhead projectors are easy to use and if not working, the most likely problem is that the bulb needs replacing as they do not like rough handling. Transparencies can be prepared in advance and used over and over again for different teaching sessions. Transparencies are reasonably cheap and easy to produce either hand written, printed from a computer, or by photocopier. Be warned, there are different types of transparency paper for different printers and photocopiers and they are not necessarily interchangeable. If a transparency melts inside a hot photocopier it is costly to repair. Do read the label on the transparency box.

Positioning

A major advantage of the OHP is that the room lights do not have to be dipped so that the teacher can see the audience to gauge student understanding. You should know your information well enough that you are able to look at the audience while occasionally glancing at the transparencies on the light box for prompting. A common mistake however is to turn away from the audience to look at the image on the wall. This will both reduce interaction and cause a problem with voice projection in a large room. Once the projector is positioned correctly, it should not be necessary to turn round to look at the image. It is however important to check that you are not obscuring the view. The image can be projected at a position over the head of the presenter in a large room but in a small room this can lead to the audience getting sore necks. For tired teachers it is one of the mediums that allows you to teach sitting down.

As you can see from point number 14 on this transparency...

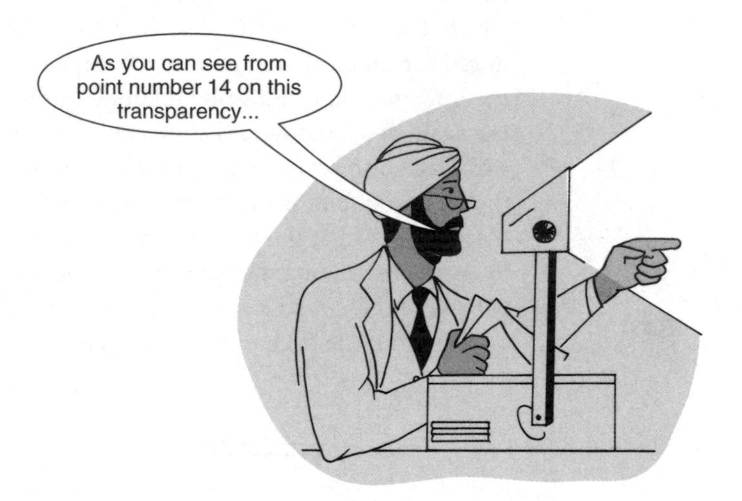

Clarity

The content of the overhead transparency is very important. Students cannot read what is on the transparency and listen at the same time, especially if what you are saying is only loosely related to the projected material. Try not to overcrowd transparencies as this will make the writing too small and time-consuming to read. If it is necessary to put a lot of information on one transparency, cover some up with a piece of paper or lay a pencil on the light source to highlight the part you are talking about, but try to avoid pointing as hand movements near the projector are greatly magnified. As a general rule, limit yourself to seven words per line, four lines per page and a minimum of 18 point font. In a smaller room try not to use the bottom third of the acetate as this section of the projected image cannot be seen by those who are not in the front row.

A great advantage of the OHP is that transparencies can be used in any order. It is easy to return to the first one without having flip through all the rest. Complex pictures can be built up in stages by overlaying up to four transparencies on one another.

One disadvantage of the OHP is that the fan makes a noise and a small room can get quite hot. To minimize this turn it off when it is not being used. It will return at the flick of a switch.

Slides

Slides produce excellent images that cannot be reproduced to the same quality by other methods (Laidlaw, 1987b). Slides are transportable, reusable, flexible, and reliable. It is most important to number slides in case of accident and also to know how to load them in a slide projector. Labelling the slides with a dot on one corner helps. Slides may be used to add realism with photographs. If professionally produced, slides can present information well and in colour. Disadvantages of slides are that they must be prepared well ahead and are inflexible once produced. They need to be projected in a darkened room.

PowerPoint

Microsoft PowerPoint is a computer presentation package. It can be used to produce presentations and handouts. The presentations can be viewed in several ways: directly on a computer, projected using a data projector, printed directly onto acetate for use with an OHP, or onto 35 mm slides by your audio-visual department. An advantage of PowerPoint is its transportability. Presentations can be saved on a floppy disc or emailed to colleagues. Presentations can even be run on computers without PowerPoint using the 'pack and go' facility or by copying the PowerPoint viewer onto a compact disc.

Producing a presentation

The software is available on most modern computers and a presentation written in PowerPoint can look very professional. Although it can initially take time to become familiar with PowerPoint, those who are computer literate should find it easy to use and could probably master the basics in around half an hour. PowerPoint can produce exciting presentations, with graphics, photographs, music clips, videos, or information from the Internet. The help menu will guide you to some extent, but to become familiar with all the facilities probably requires going on a course. It is tempting to produce very complex presentations indeed, but there are two problems. First, too many special effects may detract from the main message you are trying to get across, and secondly, complex presentations lead to large file sizes. As a result they will run very slowly or not fit on a floppy disc. Presentations in black and white with no special effects are smaller and consequently quicker.

Clarity

There are many readily prepared packages available in the PowerPoint software and these 'design templates' can be adapted to fit any presentation. If designing your own, to ensure legibility the following suggestions are made:

(a) When projecting onto a screen use at least 18 point font preferably sans serif, e.g. Arial as otherwise the tops of letters may be cut off.

(b) Dark background with light letters is better for projection but if the room is not going to be very dark it may be better to use dark lettering on a light background.

(c) If you are making OHP transparencies from a PowerPoint package it is also best to use a light background and dark letters.

Once the presentation has been written it can be easily modified. As you become more familiar with the software, you will find many useful facilities, e.g. options for hiding slides, timing a presentation (aim to allow two–three minutes per slide), and producing handouts.

Potential problems

The only real disadvantage of using PowerPoint is that as it is technology dependent it is less reliable than other more old-fashioned audio-visual methods. Save your presentation in the early (4.0) version, as it is the most likely to work on another computer. You may lose some special effects in the process, but at least you will have a presentation. Many people seem to have a problem getting the projector to work—so do try it out on location, have a back-up set of overheads or slides, or an IT expert to hand if you are not confident with the equipment.

> If you are using video clips with PowerPoint remember to use the "PACK AND GO" command when saving the presentation to CD, otherwise the video sequence will be lost.

Video

Video tapes are popular with students, as they are realistic and interesting. They are a useful way of helping students to see the whole picture and a good way to demonstrate practical skills. They can also be used very effectively as triggers to open discussions by stopping them at certain points. Video cameras can also be used to video students and provide feedback on consultation skills especially communication skills. This can be done either using simulated patient or real patients as long as consent is obtained. Although initially the presence of a camera may interfere with the process, video can be an excellent eye opener.

There are a variety of ready-made commercial videos that are available for use in teaching. Whilst some of these are excellent, some will be irrelevant to your own aims and objectives and therefore all commercially produced videos require assessment before use. Most institutions have their own video cameras and it is now possible to produce material that can be tailor-made. Having said this, to produce a high quality video tape can require considerable expertise and time (Stewart, 2001).

Video conferencing and live video lecturing are other newly available technologies enabling people to be brought together across different sites. They can be a time and money saving option in the long run as it means people do not have to physically travel.

> Medical videos can be borrowed from the British Medical Association library by BMA members. For a list of titles Tel: 0207 383 6625.

Advantages and disadvantages of different AV aids

	Advantages	Disadvantages
Black board/ white board	Flexible and cheap.	Need to have clear writing.
	Good for brainstorming or evolving ideas.	Not permanent.
	Can involve the student.	For small audiences only.

Flip chart	Flexible and relatively cheap. Good for brainstorming or evolving ideas. Can involve the student. Ideas can be written in advance and stored.	Need to have clear writing. Cumbersome and difficult to store. For small audiences only.
OHP	Readily available. Low maintenance. Produce overheads in advance and reuse. Use overheads in any order.	Poor for large audiences. Need care to ensure legibility.
Slides	Projectors readily available. Can be used flexibly. Good reproduction of photographs.	Prepared in advance. Room needs to be dark.
Video	Interesting and motivating. Shows real clinical material. Wide range of videos available. Invaluable for consultation skills.	Equipment often stolen. Expensive. Time-consuming to make new videos.
PowerPoint	Looks professional. Relatively easy to produce and modify at short notice. Can be used to produce slides and OHPs. Can incorporate video/photos/music.	Expensive. Technology dependent Needs dark room. Special effects can distract from the main message.

Handouts and study guides

'What is written without effort is in general read without pleasure'.

– Dr Johnson

Despite great advances in technology, paper is still the easiest method of distributing information. Handouts are a very common way to supplement a teaching session, but to be of any value, they must be read. All too often handouts that are painstakingly produced are found discarded at the end of a session. In order to avoid this, try to ensure handouts are helpful by considering their purpose, their content, their design, and when they are distributed.

Study guides are designed to help students learn. They often accompany a course, and show the students how they can make the most of the learning opportunities on the course. The best study guides incorporate self-tests for the students to monitor their learning, and encourage active learning (Laidlaw and Harden, 1990).

Purpose

It is worth thinking about what you are trying to achieve with your handouts. Are my handouts designed to prepare students for a session, to complement the teaching, or to outline further reading? What your handouts are for will determine when and how you use them.

Prior to teaching:

- To standardize prior knowledge.
- To act as a schema activator.

During teaching:

- To guide students through a teaching session.
- To aid interaction.
- To emphasize or summarize the main points.

After teaching:

- To emphasize or summarize the main points.
- To reinforce learning.
- To amplify the content.

Content

To act as a schema activator or standardize knowledge students must read the handout before the session. This means you must ensure that they are distributed in time. To maximize the number of students that read them, make them short with concise information arranged logically. Keep the content relevant and interesting, and consider including a task (e.g. a self-test) or group activity to encourage students to think and 'discover for themselves'.

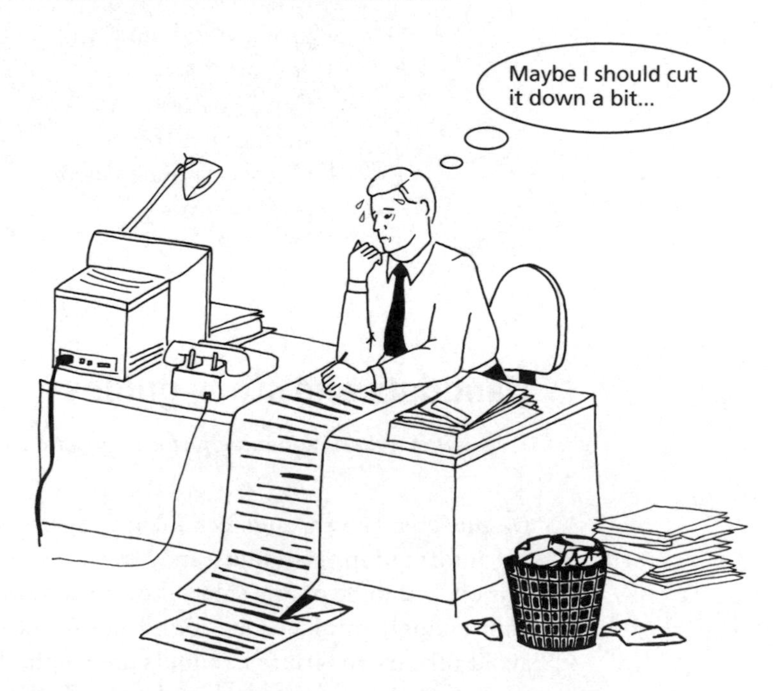

Design

Attention grabbing handouts are more likely to be read. Whatever you include in the handout, layout must be considered. With modern computer packages handouts are easy to produce—but this may mean students receive more and more handouts. Make sure yours stand out.

Having considered the purpose and content of the handout, consider the layout. Layout is very important as students may be put off by pages and pages of text.

Ensure the handout is legible by using standard font such as Times New Roman and that the print is large enough—point 12 as a minimum. Leave sizeable spaces for annotation to enable students to individualize copies and make them relevant. Break up text to stimulate interest by the use of clear headings, bold, italics, or capitals. Highlight important points by use of colour, bullet points, or symbols. Reinforce learning by use of pictures, think points, and breaks for activity. If making copies of handouts, check that the photocopier has not chopped off the edges or made the print too faint to read.

Distribution

To guide students through a teaching session and aid interaction it must be remembered that students cannot read and listen at the same time. If handouts are to be used during a teaching session, distribute them at the point in the session for which they are relevant. Build in time for the handouts to be both distributed and read. For a large group of students enlist student help in the distribution. If the handout is to explain a complicated diagram, etc. hand it out just before you want to discuss it, make sure that all the students have a copy, and give students time to study it. Do not start talking again until all the students have read it. If the handout is to guide students through a teaching session, consider using headings or a skeleton leaving enough space for students notes and annotations.

Unless it is very close to an exam when motivation and anxiety is running high, handouts given at the end may never be read. If planning to give handouts at the end, tell students this is the case and be explicit about what the content is. If designed to act as a summary the handout should be directly related to the teaching session and contain the key points but no new information. If designed to reinforce learning, you could include self-test opportunities or an assignment. If the handout is designed to amplify information this should be made clear. If it contains references or suggestions for further reading state whether this is optional or additional information rather than a summary. Do not use the handout as a reward for staying to the end of a lecture—the lecture should be good enough to attend.

PowerPoint can be used to produce handouts directly related to slides.

Computer-assisted learning (CAL)

Computers are now widespread and cheap. All medical students and teachers will have access to a computer and many will have their own. Computer-assisted learning is seen as a possible solution to many of the problems caused by increasing student numbers, as it has the potential to deliver high quality teaching to a large number of students at (relatively) low cost.

Guidelines for the use of computers in medical education have been produced by the World Federation for Medical Education (1994). Its recommendations are that computers should be integrated into the medical undergraduate curriculum and that access to computers, the World Wide Web, and email should be improved.

It appears there is enthusiasm for using information and communication technology in medical education (Slotte *et al.*, 2001). It should not be assumed however that just because it is new it is better (Vichitvejpaisal *et al.*, 2001).

Although most students now enter medical school equipped with some IT knowledge there is growing recognition of the need for greater computer literacy. Medical students need to be prepared to work in a medical setting which is becoming increasingly reliant upon computer technology (Koschmann, 1995).

CAL enables learners to set their own pace and is superb for action demonstrations, simulations, and for problem-based activities offering instant feedback. Interaction can be built into programmes to allow self-test opportunities at intervals and hyperlinks can allows students to follow an individual path through the information.

You can make your own CAL programmes with the help of your audio-visual department (Hamilton *et al.*, 1999). These can be of very high quality but the process is time-consuming and expensive. If you do decide to produce your own, use a teaching style which is familiar to your students and remember to KISS (keep it simple silly). CAL also requires ongoing expertise as new problems arise, and information, software, and hardware require updating. This makes it costly to maintain.

It is important to remember that using this sort of software is to facilitate learning rather than display one's own technical skills.

CD-ROM

A CD-ROM (compact disc read only memory) is a type of electronic text book with associated learning activities. You may have already tried some of the commercially produced packages but just as with video you will need to assess each one before use. As digital video compressing improves, an increasing amount of text, graphics, and even full motion video can now be displayed on CD-ROM. In order to be most effective, students must have clear guidance as to the aims and objectives of the programme and be provided with appropriate feedback.

Web-based learning

Web-based or Internet-based learning simply means learning that uses the Internet. This can be at its most basic level use of materials found on the Web just as one would use a library or any other resource the only difference being searching for it on the Web. A more technological use could be learning in a 'Web-based classroom'.

Web-based materials

There is an almost infinite amount of information available on the Web. There are two major problems with this information. First, it is not peer reviewed so attention must be paid that the quality is of a sufficiently high standard for your own purposes. Secondly, Internet search engines are far less specific and sensitive compared with those used to search medical literature for example Medline (e.g. Ovid or WinSpirs) thus resulting in a large number of 'hits'. You and your students may need some initial training in how to search the Web efficiently and assess information. As a teacher you can avoid these problems by designing Web-based materials for your own students. Your institution may be able to offer you some training in this.

Before you develop a Web-based session think about whether it will be suitable for your topic and your students. Would it be easier for them to access the information in another way (i.e. using textbooks or Medline)? Do you have the facilities for students to be able to access the technology and the technical ability to help them when they get stuck? Remember that you will need to factor in initial training for students and tutors but also ongoing technical, administrative, and educational support.

The Web-based classroom

This is a form of distance learning which enables tutors and students geographically separated to come together in a virtual classroom (Palloff and Pratt, 2001). Distance learning can be impersonal and isolating for students and courses designed this way may suffer from high drop-out rates. The key to success is interactivity. Just as in face to face teaching, it is helpful if interaction is initially fostered by the tutor and just as with the setting up of any group it is important to set ground rules. It is also the role of the tutor to act as moderator to ensure that ground rules are obeyed. In order to be able to do this effectively, tutors need training and support (Salmon and Page, 2000). There are two main types of online interaction: synchronous where course participants come together at a certain time and 'talk' online, or asynchronous where students place items on a notice board to be read by others. It is also nice for students to have the opportunity to talk online in private (rather like a student bar) and the tutor would not normally enter unless invited. Facilities such as a virtual library and debating chamber can also be built in. To enable interactivity online, specific software is needed. There are a number of commercially available packages which enable interactivity to assist with production of Web-based applications courses, e.g. www.blackboard.com, www.webct.com, www.embanet.com. At the time of going to press these are available however it is a fast moving world out there!

Although novel and attractive, being technology dependent means it is expensive and can, without appropriate support, be unreliable, but these modern approaches can add interest.

The key to a successful online classroom is not content but interactivity.

Summary

Teaching materials should enhance the learning in your sessions. There are a variety of materials that you can use.

'Chalk and talk' is cheap, flexible, and requires little equipment. It is good for evolving themes or for 'brainstorming exercises'. OHPs are cheap and easy to produce, provide flexibility in sequencing, good audience participation, and ability to build up complex ideas in stages as a session progresses. PowerPoint looks professional, it is cheap once initial outlay has been made for computer, versatile, portable, and easily modified.

Video is flexible, realistic, and allows a novel approach to learning. It can be a powerful tool for learning clinical skills, communication skills, and can also be used for assessment. Handouts are portable, require no additional equipment for use by the learner, and can be from a number of sources.

Sophisticated CAL packages and Web-based applications can be interesting and interactive. Students can receive immediate feedback on progress in self-tests. There are excellent packages and Web sites available, some free on the Internet, but every commercially available package needs to be extensively reviewed by the teacher.

Conclusion

Modern technology means that a range of teaching materials can be made available at reasonable cost even to a small teaching institution. It can be seen however that, although modern technologies make it easier to make lessons fun, old-fashioned methods can be used in different ways to ensure lessons are interactive and interesting. In order to facilitate students to learn and get the most out of the course, it is important to be aware of the range of facilities available and to have a knowledge of their use.

Whether you are producing the most simple of blackboard diagrams or the most high-tech computer package there are some basic principles for maximizing effectiveness.

Maximizing effectiveness of audio-visual aids

1. Relevance to the purpose and for the level of the student ability.
2. Linkage to existing knowledge and the rest of the learning activity.
3. Simplicity of language and design.
4. Emphasize signposting of important ideas, key facts, etc.
5. Consistency within a particular package, and if possible across your department packages, to enable students to get a feel for what is expected of them and how to best use the resource.

References

Ausubel, D. P., Novak, J. S., and Hanesian, H. (1978) *Educational psychology: a cognitive view*, 2nd edn. New York: Holt, Rinehart and Winston.

Gagné, R., Briggs, L., and Wager, W. (1988) *Principles of instructional design*, 3rd edn. New York: Holt, Rinehart and Winston.

Hamilton, N. M., Furnace, J., Duguid, K. P., Helms, P. J., and Simpson, J. G. (1999) Development and integration of CAL: a case study in medicine. *Med Educ* **33**, 298–305.

Koschmann, T. (1995) Medical education and computer literacy: learning about, through, and with computers. *Acad Med* **70**, 818–21.

Laidlaw, J. M. (1987a) Twelve tips for the users of the overhead projector. *Med Teach* **9**, 247–51.

Laidlaw, J. M. (1987b) Twelve tips on preparing 35 mm slides. *Med Teach* **9**, 389–93.

Laidlaw, J. M. (1995) *Principles of learning: IMD2*. Dundee: Centre for Medical Education.

Laidlaw, J. M., and Harden, R. M. (1990) What is . . . a study guide? *Med Teach* **12**, 7–12.

Palloff, M. R., and Pratt, K. (2001) Lessons from the Cyberspace classroom the realities of on line teaching. San Francisco: Jossey Bass.

Rumelhart, D. E. (1980) Schemata: the building blocks of cognition. In *Theoretical issues in reading comprehension* (ed. R. J. Spiro, B. C. Bruce, and W. F. Brewer), pp. 33–58. Hillsdale, NJ: Lawrence Erlbaum Associates.

Salmon, G., and Page, K. (2000) E-Moderating: The key to teaching and learning online. London: Kogan Page.

Slotte, V., Wangel, M., and Lonka, K. (2001) Information technology in medical education: a nationwide project on the opportunities of the new technology. *Med Educ* **35**, 990–5.

Stewart, A. (2001) Audio and video recordings. In *A practical guide for medical teachers* (ed. J. A. Dent and R. Harden). Edinburgh: Churchill Livingstone.

Vichitvejpaisal, P., Sitthikongsak, S., Preechakoon, B., Kraiprasit, K., Parakkamodom, S., Manon, C., *et al.* (2001) Does computer-assisted instruction really help to improve the learning process? *Med Educ* **35**, 983–9.

World Federation for Medical Education. (1994) Proceedings of the World Summit on medical education. *Med Educ* **28**,

Further reading

Gibbs, G., and Habeshaw, T. (1989) Using visual aids. In *Preparing to teach: an introduction to effective teaching in higher education*, Chapter 5. TES, Bristol.

Newble, D., and Cannon, R. (1994) Preparing teaching materials and using teaching aids. In *A handbook for medical teachers*, 3rd edn, Chapter 8. Kluwer Academic Publishers, Lancaster, UK.

Quality on the line, benchmarks for success in Internet-based distance education. (2000) The Institute for Higher Education Policy, Washington DC, USA, April.

Acknowledgement

Many thanks to Dr. Geoff Wong for his contribution to this chapter.

CHAPTER 7
Teaching different group sizes

When you are initially planning your session you will have thought about the number of students you will be teaching. This will be a key factor in deciding the objectives you might be able to achieve, the teaching methods you will use, and how you might check whether learning has happened. There are three group sizes that you are likely to encounter while teaching medicine: one to one teaching, small group teaching, and lecturing to large groups. While you need your generic teaching skills in any situation, there are specific skills for managing different group sizes, which will be looked at in depth in this chapter.

One to one teaching

There are many situations in medicine where teaching and learning occur in a one to one setting. Medicine was once taught almost entirely by one to one apprenticeship, and it is still used by general practitioners and hospital doctors particularly in clinics, theatre, and on call. Some types of teaching are more successful than others in the one to one setting. You will find that teaching a clinical skill, teaching clinical reasoning, and mentoring or academic supervision all work well with one student. However exploring attitudinal issues or controversial issues where a variety of ideas and perspectives need to be explored can be difficult with only two viewpoints. While one to one teaching can be a great opportunity for a learner, it can also be an overwhelming experience. Try to set a positive mood and an educational climate that will foster learning.

One to one clinical teaching

A lot of clinical teaching takes place in small groups. However there are many times when the teacher is teaching just one student. This may be for a few minutes, for a whole clinic, surgery, or list, or for a whole day such as when students are shadowing doctors on call. Vast chunks of this education is opportunistic or 'on the hoof'. This sort of teaching is often rich and memorable because it is learning in *context* and is personalized to the learner. However, such teaching can often be less useful than it might be because it lacks structure, is often not linked to objectives, and is patchy: covering some areas in more depth than is useful and ignoring other areas completely. Usually to make up for these deficiencies such teaching is supplemented by lectures or tutorials but there are techniques that can be used that make these valuable moments of one to one teaching more structured and systematic. This makes the teaching not just more effective but more efficient which is also important in the busy clinical environment.

Techniques that can be used to make one to one clinical teaching more effective include needs assessment, keeping log books, and using the 'clinical teaching' model

(Cox, 1993) described in Chapter 8 to structure the teaching. All of these techniques are covered in more detail in Chapter 8. A few key ideas regarding these techniques are included here.

Needs assessment

Spending some time with a student to find out what they already know and what they would like to learn is vital, and easy in one to one teaching. You will then be able to pitch your teaching at the right level, focus on areas of weakness, and identify 'triggers' for teaching. An example might be teaching in a busy sexual health clinic. The student may have sat in on countless clinics before and have passed lots of speculae but never spent much time talking to patients himself and not know much about contact tracing. Having found this out, during the clinic specific patients can be identified for the student to interview. If a patient arrives with whom the issue of contact tracing is important, the teacher and student can see this patient together and this experience can be used as the 'trigger' to begin a short focused learning episode about contact tracing.

Keeping logbooks

Finding out what your student has been doing is improved by keeping an ongoing record of achievements and needs. A log can be a formal book where teacher and student record all key learning experiences during a course or a more informal record of achievements and planned learning. With one to one teaching, you can personalize logbook, learning objectives, and teaching plans to the needs of the student. If the student highlighted above moved on to his gynaecology attachment he may feel his needs are not met by performing, and being signed up for, ten more speculum examinations. Instead, you might spend some time at the beginning of the attachments finding out what he needs to know and personalizing his logbook. This would only take a few minutes and would then make the majority of teaching sessions useful for the learner.

Using set, body, and closure in all teaching sessions

In a one to one setting it is easy to think of teaching as a 'little chat' and forget to apply the set, body, closure principle, which make learning more effective. It may seem a little contrived but outlining what you are planning to achieve and why and how you are going to get there, will be a useful structure for both of you. A sense of closure and reflection about what has been achieved can be added briefly at the end of each new learning episode or at the end of a series of experiences: e.g. the end of the clinic or course.

Plan–experience–reflect

Much clinical teaching focuses on the exposure or experiences of learners. You will maximize learning if you encourage your students to spend time planning for, and reflecting on, their experiences. Use some of your time to help them with this, as it will enrich their bedside experience. In the planning stage try thinking together about the task to be performed, identify previously experienced difficulties, or explore expected difficulties. Help your student to see links between what he is about to experience and previous learning. In the reflection stage encourage your student to articulate both achievements and deficiencies, to identify why difficulties arose, and to begin to plan for the next experience.

Remember that one to one experiences can be intimidating or even overwhelming for a student, especially at the beginning of their clinical course. If you can make a special effort to make them feel comfortable and valued, they will be able to make the most of their time with you.

Academic supervision and personal tutors

These activities do not always spring to mind as 'teaching' but of course they are as they facilitate learning. Within medical education the boundaries between educational supervisors, personal tutors, and mentors are often blurred. There is a lot of confusion among students, teachers, and even institutions about what these various roles entail and often one person fulfils more than one role. Sometimes this is entirely logical and workable but sometimes it is not. In general terms a personal tutor or supervisor supports the learner and his or her learning in a broadest sense (rather than extend or deepen the academic understanding of the learner).

Usually these roles are allocated formally but often tutors slip into these roles unofficially because of relationships that have built up with students. Effective tutors/supervisors are committed to the process and have a real interest in helping students to succeed. Most importantly they have taken steps to understand their role and how that fits in with other student support systems.

As a personal tutor or academic supervisor you might have a variety of roles. You may be there purely for academic support, guiding the student through a course or curriculum. In addition, you may have an administrative or resource–provision role; guiding students to information and resources they may need. Some of you will also have a professional or career guidance role advising on professional behaviours and attitudes, job opportunities, or career pathways. Whether you are expected to or not, most will also develop a personal support role. This can be comfortable and beneficial to the student but can sometimes put you in a difficult position. If you uncover serious personal or professional issues, they will probably need to be referred on to other support services. Because the job is so complex, to be an effective personal tutor or supervisor, you will need a variety of attributes and skills.

Attributes of an effective supervisor or personal tutor

1. Interested and committed to the process.
2. Needs to understands and respect the purpose of supervision or personal tutoring.
3. Available in terms of time and location.
4. Easily contactable in person, or by phone or email.
5. Knowledgeable about:
   The course and its requirements.
   The support systems within the organization or institution.
6. A good tutor will take the time to find out about the student, their experience, their personal and professional goals, and their learning needs.
7. Will be facilitative rather than directive. A good supervisor or tutor will help the adult learner to identify learning needs and how to achieve them.
8. Respects autonomy and confidentiality.
9. Is a good role model. A good supervisor or tutor needs to ensure that his own professional behaviour can stand up to scrutiny to ensure he is a credible role model.
10. Establishes ground rules for sessions. Discusses and agrees at an early stage with the tutee about the remit of the relationship. This will also need constant reflection.
11. Encourages both reflection on the past and planning for the future.

Mentoring

Being a mentor is rather like being a personal tutor or academic supervisor. You will be expected to provide academic, personal, and professional support in the same way as an effective personal tutor or supervisor. However in a mentoring relationship there is more emphasis on personal support alongside academic support. So how can we become good mentors? The Homeric concept of the mentor being a wise counsellor, a good friend, and a role model encapsulates the key prerequisites of a good mentor. You will need to be in some way wise: this can range from simply being in a more senior position to being a perceived expert in their field. You will need to be a good counsellor with good communication skills and access to information about support systems, training, and advice that is available. Finally you will need to be a friend, someone with whom one can share failures as well as successes. Mentoring is discussed in more detail in Chapter 12.

Learning and teaching in small groups

For practical reasons medical students are often taught in groups such as tutorial groups or 'firms'. Good small group teaching encourages self-directed learning, problem or task oriented learning, and learning through curiosity. It can be one of the most effective and flexible teaching methods and very rewarding for the teacher. The benefits of small group work can be maximized by making the most of the strengths of working with groups, by matching the activity and methods used in the group to the objectives for the session, and by paying attention to group management.

What do we mean by a small group?

More than one student and less than the whole year group! The size of the group that we teach is usually determined by external issues such as curriculum demands. However a group larger than about 16 students will have some difficulty in performing effectively as a group unless the tutor is in some way able to break this larger group into a series of smaller groups. The number of students in the group is not key to defining what a small group is. More important are the features that define small group learning. These have been defined as (Crosby, 1997):

- active participation
- interactive
- task oriented
- involving reflection

These are the characteristics of good small group learning. We have all been to many small group sessions where in fact none of these characteristics have been present and it is really a mini lecture given to a rather small audience. Remember that if you are planning small group work these features are what your session should be based on.

Why use small groups?

Small group learning can achieve a wide range of learning objectives. Not only are groups good places to learn knowledge, skills, and attitudes, but they allow students to develop a range of collaborative and interactive skills, which cannot be developed in one to one or large group settings. These generic skills are an important part of professional development but are frequently overlooked by the curriculum aims. Small groups also have a social role in large medical schools where small group work provides important contacts with peer and tutors.

Learning encouraged by small group working

Higher level skills

Self-directed and self-motivated learning.

Learning for understanding.

Reasoning.

Developing and defending arguments.

Problem solving.

Development of attitudes.

Generic skills

Group working.

Managing and organizing tasks.

Interpersonal skills and communicating effectively.

Presentation skills.

When should we use small groups?

Small group teaching is just one of a number of effective teaching methods we can adopt. It is not the solution for all types of teaching and sometimes it is impractical or unsuitable for the learning objectives. Small group sessions can be run in a number of ways depending on the objectives for the session, but below are a number of methods and settings where small group work is usually suitable:

- Classical tutorials;
  - Expert teacher exploring a concept or knowledge areas with a small group of learners.
- Clinical teaching sessions;
  - Ward rounds or patient focused teaching.
  - Clinical skills sessions.
  - Community-based teaching.
- Problem-based learning.
- Task-based learning or project work.
- Workshops or discussion groups;
  - Including exploring issues or producing protocols or consensus.
- Communication skills teaching.
- Ethics teaching.
- Critical appraisal and evaluating evidence.

Managing a small group

Managing an active small group teaching session can be more demanding than relatively didactic sessions. Your role as the teacher is less clearly defined, you will have to deal more closely with the behaviours and personalities in the group, and you will find problem student behaviour difficult to ignore. As a small group teacher you have two roles: management of the task and maintenance of the group. This means you need a clear understanding of the activity you have planned and how to tackle it while at the same time understanding and reacting to what is going on in the group.

Management of the task

For the group to function smoothly, the tasks need to be clearly defined. Not only do your students need to know what the task is, they will also want to know why it will be useful. Students will have experienced lots of different types of small group work. To avoid confusion, discuss the way in which the group will operate and what *you* will do. In some cases you will be very familiar with the content of the session, but in other cases you may not be a subject expert. While this can feel very uncomfortable, non-expert tutors do very well in small groups if they are practised in the skill of group facilitation and are familiar with the task and related learning objectives. In fact a subject expert can often hinder the ability of students to work collaboratively or independently. If you are a non-expert facilitator it may help to start with *'Hello, I am here to help you to learn about X, but I am not an expert on X, so if you have questions we will be finding out the answers together..'* or *'I'm here to help you find the answers . . .'*

Your role in task management may include opening the discussion, summarizing and clarifying, timekeeping, debriefing the group on the activity, i.e. checking and clarifying with the group what has been achieved. Remember to allow time for reflection on the task before the session ends.

Heron (1997) outlines modes of facilitation that can be adopted. A good facilitator adopts the most appropriate mode for the task. Continually operating in the same mode is frustrating for facilitator and students. The following modes of facilitation have been identified:

Hierarchical. The facilitator directs the group and leads from the front by thinking and acting on behalf of the group. This commonly happens when a group or tutor is new to small group work or where the teacher is an expert in the subject. Seating arrangements with the teacher in a dominant position can encourage this mode of facilitation.

Co-operative. The facilitator shares the power with the group. The facilitator encourages the group to become more self-directing by conferring and collaborating with the group about actions and decisions. His opinion, although influential, is considered alongside the ideas of the group. Seating in a complete circle with the teacher in the same kind of position as the learners encourages this mode. Non-expert facilitators are more likely to adopt this sort of mode of facilitation.

Autonomous. The facilitator is removed from the group giving them the freedom to do things their own way. This requires careful observation and monitoring of the group to ensure the climate is right for self-determination of their learning. Allowing the group to sit in a circle with you sitting outside the circle encourages this mode.

Heron also outlines some dimensions of facilitation style or the strategies and behaviours adopted by the facilitator in a small group setting. These dimensions describe areas such the degree of directiveness, confrontation, or how interpretation is used during discussions. The facilitator style self-assessment grid is available opposite, and will enable you to identify your style and encourage facilitator development.

Facilitator style self-assessment grid

Name ____________________

John Heron in *Dimensions of facilitator style* (1977) describes the following dimensions, which are useful in determining your personal facilitator style.

Directive the facilitator clearly directs the group	*or*	**Non-directive** the facilitator encourages the group to make decisions for itself
Interpretative the facilitator offers the group interpretations of its behaviour	*or*	**Non-interpretative** the facilitator encourages the group to interpret its own behaviour
Confronting the facilitator interrupts rigid repetitive group behaviour	*or*	**Non-confronting** the facilitator encourages the group to confront itself or each other
Cathartic the facilitator encourages release of emotions in the group	*or*	**Non-cathartic** the facilitator steers the group into less emotional territory
Structuring the facilitator uses a variety of procedures to bring structure to the group	*or*	**Non-structuring** the facilitator works with the group in a relatively unstructured way
Disclosing the facilitator shares their thoughts, feelings, and experiences with the group	*or*	**Non-disclosing** the facilitator keeps their own thoughts, feelings, and experience to themselves, and plays a neutral role

Please rate yourself as a group facilitator as you are now by marking an appropriate point along each dimension below. There is no objective right or wrong position.

Directive ____ Non-directive

Interpretative ____ Non-interpretative

Confronting ____ Non-confronting

Cathartic ____ Non-cathartic

Structuring ____ Non-structuring

Disclosing ____ Non-disclosing

You may also wish to consider where you would like to be along each dimension and how you might achieve this move.

Maintenance of the group

This is sometimes referred to as group facilitation. Facilitation is defined as 'to make a task easier to accomplish'. In teaching terms facilitation means helping learners to achieve a task where the prime responsibility for learning rests within the group and only secondarily with the teacher. Thus a facilitator is helping the learner to be more self-reliant. This rather 'hands-off' mode of teaching takes some getting used to both for the teacher and the learner, and it is worth being explicit with learners about the role you plan to adopt.

One of your key roles will be getting students to participate. Try using non-verbal prompts and silence to encourage students to expand on an idea or suggestion. Phrases such as '*Would you like to tell us more about your idea.. . . .*' '*That is an interesting question, what do the rest of the group think?*' and '*Do any of you feel there might be an alternative explanation here. . . . ?*' are useful when you wish to deflect the discussion back into the group. Try to keep your own value judgements to yourself as they can be inhibiting to the group and instead try to use the group to refute controversial statements. Participation, even for quieter members, is made easier if your group of students often work together. If this is the case, then they will become quite close. This will allows students to develop the confidence to discuss difficult issues, and confront difficult areas. Encourage this and allow students the time they need for discussion among themselves; remember that peer learning is highly effective.

Maintaining a group

1. Be aware of your role as a facilitator, rather than a content expert.
2. Clarify your role in the group.
3. Participation—try to encourage students to talk and interact with each other and with you.
4. Encourage bonding among the group members.
5. Value the team-work aspect of the group work as a useful generic competence. Reflect this back to the group from time to time especially if things are going very well or rather badly.
6. Be aware that you may unexpectedly take on an informal pastoral care role, and if this is uncomfortable, be aware of the support systems you can direct students to.

How to set up an effective small group

If you want your small group to run well, you need to get the atmosphere right for learning, help to form the group, and be clear about the tasks to be performed and the strategies to be used. You may need to break the group down into subgroups to share out tasks so they can be achieved within a reasonable time frame.

Getting the setting right

Seating is an important factor in small group work. A lecture theatre set up with the chairs in rows does not lend itself to small group work. If the furniture moves then move it! If it does not you may need to get students sitting on desks to form some kind of circle. A horseshoe will encourage a hierarchical set-up with the teacher in control. A circular arrangement encourages a more inclusive atmosphere with all participants equally able to join in and to take turns. It also suggests a more flexible role for the teacher.

Ground rules

To work together well your students need to feel comfortable and safe. You can do this by making sure that the group know what to expect and by agreeing ground rules. Although this is time-consuming, it is vital for all small group work. Ground rules outline the acceptable behaviour and boundaries in the group, and tell students what they can expect from you and each other. They usually include a requirement for confidentially and rules about participation and turn taking. No one set of ground rules will work for every group in every situation, and so the group as a whole should set them. Remember to review the ground rules as the group works and matures.

Sample ground rules for a series of small group sessions

- All participants have a right to have their views heard.
- All participants will make an effort to be an active participant.
- Shirking or slacking will be challenged by other group members if it is impacting on the group task.
- The group members will rotate through the following roles: Timekeeper, Chair, and Scribe.
- Issues discussed within the group will remain confidential to the group.
- Challenges or argument are encouraged but they must be constructive.
- The group will review the group *process* as well as the group *progress* with the task in hand at regular intervals.
- Feedback will be given using the following rules:
  Subject before observer.
  Positive before negative.
  Behaviour not person.
  Specific not general.
  Negative comments will be accompanied by ways to improve.

The format of the group

The way the group is formed may be outside your control. Your group may be some random allocation or a pre-existing group such as a 'firm' or tutorial group. The dynamics of a group can vary dramatically depending on how it was formed, i.e. who the participants are, their relationships with each other, and whether the members have had experiences of past group work within this particular group. It is worth spending some time finding out the extent to which the group knows each other and their past group experiences. Groups particularly appreciate some attention to what they feel has worked well in the past and what they have not found useful.

Breaking the group into subgroups

Unless you are working with the smallest of groups, at times your small group will need splitting up into smaller groupings to work effectively. Think about how you split the group up as it may have an impact on how these subgroups perform. Try to encourage students to work with different people on different tasks rather than just with their friends. This encourages collaborative working and exposes students to new ideas and attitudes.

There are a number of ways of forming subgroups to favour the tasks you hope to achieve. Race and Brown (1998) outline the following formats and their relative strengths and weaknesses:

Random groups. Participants are randomly allocated to a small group without prior knowledge of working with each other. Group dynamics can be a problem as strong members struggle for power and conflicts occur. Lazy or non-participatory members can blend into the background.

Rotating syndicates. Students are grouped systematically for each task. The teacher determines who is in each group and individuals are constantly introduced to working with new group members. Encourages good group working skills and spreads difficult, uncooperative, or dominant students around the group so the same people do not always get lumbered. Also a useful format if groups are going to be assessed on group work.

Friendship groups. Students choose who they work with. Students like this format but it doesn't foster peers supporting each other. Students seek out like-minded individuals with the more able students clumping together. Not good if you are assessing group work as one group will always be more able than the other groups.

Hybrid groups. Students choose one friend they would like to work with and these pairs are randomly mixed to form groups. Perhaps the best of both worlds but a tendency for the pairs to work in isolation.

Learning teams. The teacher specifically forms the group with the individuals' strengths and weaknesses in mind.

Ice-breakers

In the early stage of small group work it can be difficult to get the students working as a group. This is particularly the case if the don't know each other or are unfamiliar with small group work. This is a natural stage of group work (see *Life cycle of a group*). You can encourage the group to start to interact with each other by using ice-breakers. These are simply exercises designed to be fun and interactive and by being related to personal details, encourage engagement between members of the group. A simple ice-breaker might be '*Turn to the person next to you and discuss what you hope to get out of this session*' or '*I would like you to tell the group your name and one interesting fact about you that people might not guess just by looking at you . . .*' More elaborate ice-breakers might be for example, a version of the following: A member of the group gives their name. The next person needs to give the name of the person before then add their name to the list and so on until the last person in the group will have to list all the names in order. Remember these exercises are supposed to be fun and easy for people to participate in.

Some small group teaching methods

There is a wide range of teaching methods that can be successfully used in the small group setting. The methods you use will be determined by both the task and the objectives you are hoping to achieve.

Tutorials

These sessions typically involve a small group and a subject expert teacher. Tutorials let students critically investigate and probe material and clarify and build on their learning in a given area. For a tutorial to work well, you should expect the students to have prepared the material in advance, and be ready to discuss it. If your students have not prepared or you are uncomfortable with small group work, then there is a danger that the tutorial will deteriorate into a small group lecture. Because tutorials are often teacher-led, the areas covered may be patchy and narrow.

You need both content expertise and facilitation skills to run a tutorial. Try encouraging a format where the learners provide the structure, generate and answer questions, and test out options and hypotheses. Your role will be to give input when requested or where clarification is needed.

Because tutorials depend on students having prepared the work, they are hampered by some, or less frequently all, of the students arriving unprepared. Tutorials therefore need some attention to ground rules. Ensure students know that they must take responsibility for preparing for the session and that they know and expect that they will be in the driving seat. In return your commitment to the group could be to give input if and when it is required and to give feedback on performance.

Seminars

Like tutorials, the emphasis of seminars is preparation by the learners. Seminars are classically about learners preparing and presenting a piece of work. The task or project may be assigned and prepared during the same session as the presentation component or may be done in a separate session. Some or all students do the presentation and all students then discuss and evaluate the materials presented. Seminars promote research ability, critical thinking, discussion, group leadership, and presentation skills. It is best if all students are encouraged to prepare the material rather than just those who will present it.

During the preparation stage try to offer suggestions and support to the seminar leaders and make sure that the same students don't always end up presenting. The group should understand that everyone is expected to contribute and, time allowing, you will expect everyone to present at some point. During the session you should encourage discussion and if appropriate probe both the presenters and the rest of the group for understanding. Constructive feedback on both the content of the presentation and the presentation skills is important, and should come from you and the group.

One of the benefits of seminars is the chance for the student presenter to lead the session. Try to overcome all temptations or encouragement to take over. Try sitting amongst the students and try to keep silent unless invited to contribute. If a presenter gets seriously stuck do enough to get them back on the right track and then encourage them to continue.

Problem-based learning (PBL)

This describes a learning method where a problem is the focus for generating and achieving learning objectives. It is highly suitable for small group learning and is discussed in depth in Chapter 5.

Free discussion groups

Students will usually love or loathe free discussion and brainstorming. Badly planned unstructured discussion or brainstorming sessions deliver 'pointless' teaching where students don't feel they have learned anything at all and are completely turned off. Free discussion does not mean 'free for all'. If well planned and run, these sessions can generate animated participation and can be great fun and great learning at the same time.

Free discussion groups are useful for addressing controversial or sensitive issues. Consider using a clinical scenario, press cutting, or some data as stimulus material to set the students off. You need to introduce the material, facilitate and mediate the discussion, and finally summarize the discussion. With complex issues there may be no clear answers, leading to participants being more confused at the end of the session than at the outset. Planning at the outset for this outcome and acknowledgement of these feelings is helpful and gives the activity more meaning.

Brainstorming

Brainstorming is a useful technique where creative solutions to problems or scenarios are being sought. You can use it at the start of other methods such as PBL or use it as the teaching technique for the whole session. Again the session needs some structure to maintain attention to the task. There is a simple three step sequence to brainstorming activities: generate ideas, clarify ideas, evaluate ideas. Gibbs and Habeshaw (1989) suggest three ground rules for the first stage of brainstorming:

- Call out suggestions in any order.
- Don't explain or justify your suggestions.
- Don't comment on other people's suggestions.

These ground rules ensure that group members have freedom to express their ideas. In this first stage it is worth clarifying that all ideas are welcome and that you expect everyone to contribute something and that you will only continue the process until no new ideas are being generated. If people are reluctant to speak up, i.e. if they think their ideas are too controversial, you can encourage learners to write down their thoughts on a 'Post-it' note and collect and collate them anonymously. At this first stage it is important to write down *all* the suggestions or ideas generated. This is usually best on a flip chart or white board.

Once ideas have been generated the group needs to work to clarify and group the ideas and suggestions. These ideas or themes are then explored one by one and the merits are discussed.

Role play

Role play is useful in sessions that explore attitudes and behaviours, and excellent for learning communication skills. Usually volunteers (or conscripts!) enact a scenario you have outlined. This allows students to rehearse difficult clinical situations in relative safety and gain some insight into how patients feel (by playing the part of the patient). However the plan is not just to have a vivid experience but to reflect upon it and learn from it. Role play sessions require the following elements;

(a) *Setting the scene.* Discuss the nature of the session and the planned learning objectives. Students need a clear understanding of the purpose or the role play, their individual roles in the session, and the procedure, for example whether video will be used.

(b) *A scenario.* Start off with a well planned scenario but allow your students to try different scenarios once they get started. Giving specific roles to the observers is useful for the debriefing section. For example ask one student to comment on what was said, another on non-verbal communication, etc.

(c) *Debriefing.* Get your students to think about and discuss their experiences. Debriefing is especially important if the role play has been emotionally charged or if the role play demanded students to behave towards each other in an uncharacteristic way such as displaying aggression. This debrief may need to be a group activity or a moment of personal quiet time. Also it is important to keep all feedback constructive.

Students are often reluctant to take part in role play but afterwards say that it was a very useful experience. The term 'role play' has a bad press with some students who complain about it not being 'real'. To counter this you could not mention the words 'role play' at all and instead refer to the exercise as 'practising' what they have just learnt (e.g. '*Today we will look at breaking bad news, and putting into practice some of the suggestions made by the group . . .*'). As the purpose of role play is to simulate reality, so that students learn in context, make your scenarios as realistic as possible. Try to base the work around a real experience or scenario.

Your ground rules may need to negotiate the level at which individuals take part. Some students' learning style means they will always be the volunteer and others the natural observer. Decide in advance if you are happy for students to choose the roles they prefer or if it is important that everyone has a go. The safety and confidentiality within the group may need to be restated.

Skills training

Like role play, skills training helps learners to develop experiential understanding. It allows students to practise and refine skills and competencies in a low risk environment. Increasingly skills training is based around skills models and computer programmes. Make sure that the task is a group task with opportunities to learn from each other and to share successes and failures. Skills training is covered in detail in Chapter 8.

Small groups and dynamics

Every individual will bring their own personality and behaviours to a group and these characteristics will have an effect on the rest of the group and on you.

In any group setting people will be constantly interacting with each other and experiencing a wide range of feelings about other members of the group. Usually this is productive and generates enthusiastic and useful team-working. Occasionally it will cause problems and stop learning from happening. Being aware of what is happening in your group is an important group maintenance task of the teacher. You may find it worthwhile to spend some time looking at how each individual interacts with the rest of the group especially if you are going to work with the same group regularly or for long periods of time.

Meredith Belbin is well known for his work on teams (Belbin, 1981). Belbin has written extensively about the various ways individuals behave in a group setting, and suggests our basic personality confers on us a set of characteristics that we will habitually display in a group setting. The Belbin test for assessing team roles is a self-perception questionnaire that can be completed by a group in about ten minutes.

The Belbin team roles

Shaper. Highly strung, outgoing, and dynamic. Can handle and thrive on confrontation. Often drive others into action. Can be impatient and offend others.

Plant. Individual, unorthodox, and creative. Inclined to disregard details or protocols.

Co-ordinator. Controlled, tackles problems calmly, welcoming all contributions without losing sight of objectives. Can clash with shapers.

Monitor evaluator. Serious minded and prudent. Good at weighing up pros and cons but can seems dry and lacking in ability to motivate others.

Resource investigator. Good communicators, can think on their feet and probe others for information. Liable to lose interest once initial fascination has passed.

Implementer. Well organized and systematic. Have a sense of what is feasible and relevant. Can lack flexibility and resistant to unproven ideas.

Team worker. Supportive, sociable, and promotes team spirit. Can be indecisive and fail to provide clear lead to others.

Completer finisher. Orderly and conscientious. Fulfils promises but worries about small details and reluctant to let go.

Specialist. Dedicated and single minded. Acquires skills and knowledge through sheer commitment along a narrow front but lacks interest in other people's work.

Knowledge of an individual's role allows the group to make the most of each individual's strengths. However, an effective team or group is made up of a variety of role types. This means that if a particular role type is absent, it may be necessary for someone in the group to take on this role to ensure the group functions well. It also means that if a group is made up of an excess of one or two role types (e.g. a room full of co-ordinators) it may cause problems within the group.

Dealing with problem situations in small group work

Some students love small group work and others detest it. This may be a reflection of their personal learning preferences but may also be coloured by their past experiences of group work. Poorly planned and executed small group work where the group is poorly managed and the task is inappropriate is destined to fail. When group work is not going well it is worth taking a step back and going through a checklist of possible problems. Consider not only why the problem is happening but also how it is going to be rectified. You need to decide whether to let the group realize that there is a problem or whether to bring it to their attention. Once the problem has been identified, either the group or you will have to deal with it, and this may take place either within the group or by raising the problem with the individuals concerned. It is generally most appropriate to raise the problem within the group and ask for their help in finding a solution. This is because sometimes your perceptions of the difficulty do not match that of the students. You may have come to the wrong diagnosis, or you may perceive a problem where there is not one. In some cases, a person or behaviour may have a negative impact on you, but not affect the group process or progress at all. Finally, working with students to solve problem behaviour encourages a co-operative and nurturing climate, which is a climate in which small group work thrives.

Diagnosing problems in a group

1 Have I planned the session well?

2 Is the task appropriate to small group work?

3 Have I defined the task well enough and helped the group to carry it out?

4 What am *I* doing in the group? Am I being too hands-off or too hands-on?

5 Have I spent enough time getting to know the group?

6 Have we started to veer away from our ground rules?

7 Is it just the stage the group are going through. Small groups are not static in their behaviours, but tend to follow a recognized pattern over time. They may not have reached a mature 'performing' stage yet.

8 What are individual's roles within the group. Are they hindering progress?

9 Is a group member being difficult and if so why (see below)?

Small groups are not static in their behaviours. When individuals come together to form a group the interactions in that group follow a recognized pattern over time (Tuckman, 1965). It is worth thinking about where your group is at, particularly if things are not going well. These stages can be summarized as follows.

Forming. The group is anxious, dependent on its leader, and searching for behavioural norms. At this stage the activities of the group may feel stilted and difficult to initiate.

Storming. There is internal conflict as individuals assert their positions. There will be negotiations as to who contributes what, power relationships and uncertainties about how to proceed. At this stage there may be conflict and dissent amongst the group and a lot of unconstructive bickering.

Norming. If the group survives the last phase group cohesion occurs and norms emerge. The group works constructively together to develop solutions.

Performing. Group roles are functional, flexible, and conflicts are handled so that tasks are performed efficiently. This is the most effective stage for the group to work together.

Ending. This occurs as the tasks are completed or time runs out and often focuses on sharing past experiences or attempts to hold the group together.

Dealing with a problem student in a small group

At times some individuals seem hell-bent on sabotaging a small group. This makes teachers feel very uncomfortable. You may sometimes get angry and want to deal with the problem by direct confrontation but this is rarely helpful. It may encourage further bad behaviour from the student(s) (think about an attention-seeking toddler!), it may alienate you from the rest of the group, alter the atmosphere, and it usually makes you feel bad.

There is no such thing as the typical problem student, but problem behaviours usually fall into certain types. It is worth taking time to think about the type of behaviour being exhibited, why it is happening, and the tactics you will adopt to deal with it. The most important skill in working out how to deal with the problem is the skill of *diagnosing* the problem. There may be dozens of reasons why certain behaviours are being exhibited. For example a quiet student may be not joining in because he is bored, tired, emotionally stressed, timid, unhappy with the group, you, or the content of the session, or have a reflective learning style! A few questions or picking up on non-verbal cues may help you to diagnose the problem. Once you know why the behaviour is being exhibited you can begin to tackle it.

The quiet student

May be under-confident, under-stimulated, distracted, or distressed. Quieter members can be encouraged to contribute sometimes by getting them to express their non-verbal cues, e.g. '*You look like you disagree with that . . .* '. If they are timid they may also benefit from the group being asked to do things in pairs and then asking for a spokesperson from the pairs to report back to the group.

The attention seeker/disruptive student

May be bored or enjoy being the centre of attention. He may enjoy your reactions to his behaviour. Try to respond to his behaviour in an adult fashion rather than in a parent mode. Encourage the rest of the group to participate more. In a circle, sit next to him so he is not in your direct line of view, and so cannot easily attract attention. If necessary challenge the behaviour of a disruptive student: '*When you behave like that it makes my task very difficult and the group cannot get on. Is that your intention?*'

The dominant student/knowledgeable student

Often these students are very able and crave praise. Praise the contribution and then encourage input from the rest of the group. Again you may need to sit next to him so he is not in your direct line of view or try appointing him scribe—it is difficult to write and talk at the same time. When breaking up the group for tasks try putting him with other dominant students so they cannot take over the whole session. A very knowledgeable student can be utilized as a co-tutor to help you with some of the tasks.

The joker

The joker can be a distraction but a certain amount of fun can be useful in a group setting. Ensure he does not go over the line and either offend a student or patient or disrupt the teaching. Try encouraging the group to temper rather than encourage his behaviour.

The critical/challenging student

This student may be unhappy with the course or your teaching. He may have picked up signals from other teachers or students that your contribution is not valid. This is a common experience for general practice teachers. Try to make the tasks stimulating and highlight the utility of the session. It is worth checking to see if the whole group feels the same. You may need to challenge this behaviour. Again a non-confrontational approach is best: '*You seem to be trying to tell me that this work is pointless/that you don't agree with me. Shall we talk about why you feel like this and how we can put it right?*'

Planning for a small group session

When you have developed your objectives and considered the practical constraints, like group size and room facilities, you can select the most appropriate small group methods to achieve the objectives. Like all teaching small group work needs a beginning, middle, an end, and a lesson plan. The key areas that need additional consideration are summarized below.

Planning small group teaching

Introduction

Introductions and ground rules play an important part in this section especially in a new group. Use an 'ice-breaker' to get people to participate and set ground rules.
Briefing: About the task and what students will be expected to do in the time available.

Body

Activity: Choose methods that suit the objectives, the facilities, and the group size.
Questions: Try simple opening questions to start things off and strategic questions that will help keep things moving, control the discussion, or deflect issues back to the group for consideration by other members, e.g. '*That's an interesting point, what do others think?*'
Group management: Ensure all members participate using techniques like 'buzz groups'. Refrain from passing value judgements and ask the group to discuss controversial statements.
Feedback: Give constructive feedback on learning, achievement, and group performance.

Close

Ensure participants can see relevance of the session and reinforce key learning points, especially if the session has been about exploring uncertainty or attitudinal issues.

Large groups

> *Lectures can bring a subject alive and make it more meaningful. Alternatively, they can kill it.* (Brown and Manogue, 2001)

Talking to large groups presents special challenges and makes people very anxious. The *Guinness Book of Records* suggests that the most frightening thing for the most people is standing up and talking to a large audience: this rates even higher on the 'frightening stakes' than death!

Lectures are one of the most ubiquitous forms of teaching in higher education and so most medical teachers will at some time be called upon to teach large groups. In this section we will look at how to plan for a large group session, how to structure effective lectures, and how to incorporate active learning into the large group setting.

In the current educational climate, the lecture has taken a bit of a back seat in undergraduate medical education. In the quest for reduction of content overload and the introduction of novel teaching methods the lecture programme of an undergraduate course may be limited to as little as three to four hours a week. Increasingly the lecture will be given to an enormous audience some of who may be at a distant site and linked by video or a 'live-link'. Research suggests that lectures are good for conveying knowledge or expansion on a theme. Realistically, when done well, their main strengths are to introduce a topic, to convey information, and occasionally to stimulate students interest to encourage further self-directed learning.

However generally lectures are too content dense, cover too much information, and are scheduled for longer than most people can concentrate. Lecturers tend to attempt to achieve too much in a lecture and often the audience seems uninterested and keen on the handout only. Therefore if you are asked to give a lecture you have to make a special effort to combat some of the inbuilt disadvantages of the lecture format.

Preparation and organization

Before you begin to plan a large group session there are a series of questions you should ask yourself:

- Do I want to do this?
- Is this the best format?
- Do I have enough time and resources to prepare for this?

If the answer to any or all of these questions is no then you need to seriously consider whether or not you are going to do it at all. This decision may seem be out of your hands but it is worth speaking to the course organizer about your reservations together with any suggestions about a more suitable speaker or format.

Once you have decided to go ahead, it is vital to plan the structure and content very carefully. Good lectures do not happen by chance: preparation is important. Preparation gives you more of a feeling of control at a time when you may be feeling very nervous. Good preparation should be focused so that it is efficient. Spending sleepless nights endlessly worrying about whether a session will go well is counterproductive and learning a lecture entirely by heart like a script is also unlikely to be feasible or successful. Useful planning involves the following five steps;

Planning a successful lecture

Step 1—Define the content and the audience

- Check the course aims and the aims for the lecture with the course co-ordinator.
- Check the topic, title, and objectives, and how much control you have over these.
- Find out who the audience are and what they want from the session.

Step 2—Identify the content

- Determine what content should be included and what left out.
- Think about how to make the content more interesting.
- Think about how you will engage the audience.
- Consider how will you make learning or understanding happen.
- Identify the AV aids required and find out if they available.
- Remember: you will always have too much to say (you are the expert) and you will always feel pressed for time—less is more!

Step 3—Plan the structure/organization

- Determine what will go in the beginning, middle, and end.
- Think about content structure: breaking the content into chunks and varying the stimulus. Think about how you will move between sections of the body.
- Decide what teaching methods you will use.
- What is key/what can be left out if timing is a problem?
- Where and when am I going to allow questions, and what questions are likely to be asked?
- Think about what sort of handout to produce and when it will be distributed.

Step 4—Rehearsal

- Important for timing, audibility, comprehension, and to calm your nerves.
- Use video or a trusted colleague: it needs to be said aloud.
- Think about using cue cards. Number them in case you drop them and have a spare set.
- Consider memorizing the opening and conclusion, as this is when you are nervous and this is when you have maximum attention.

Step 5—Preparation on the day

- Get there early to rearrange the room and check the audio-visual aids.
- Alter temperature/curtains/lighting if necessary.
- Trust no one but yourself to set up your equipment and ensure you have back-up if equipment fails.

This may seem like a lot to remember but the planning stage is important. A few other areas need special mention.

Interaction. It is good idea to try to introduce interaction to a large group session as it encourages active learning and varies the stimulus. It is, however, time-consuming. Make sure you have allowed time for this in your lesson plan and acknowledge this in your rehearsal. As a rough guide if a lecture is highly interactive with lots of questions and answers the content should fill no more than half of the allotted time for the body of the session.

Handouts. These have been discussed in Chapter 6. Remember that if you give out a handout at the beginning of lecture, give people time to read it. They will anyway and they will then not be concentrating on your introduction. Partial handouts are useful especially if there are complicated diagrams as part of your lecture. The handout format of PowerPoint slides makes a good partial handout. Everything on the slides is there and students can annotate them if they wish. A complete transcript of the lecture is not feasible or sensible. However, producing a concise reinforcement of the key points that you have covered verbally will encourage retention of the material.

AV aids. These need careful consideration. As their name suggests they should aid rather than distract. Think about what is most suitable and have back-up ideas for when the slide projector jams or the projector is not compatible with your laptop.

Structure and delivery of large group teaching sessions

As always a well structured teaching session has a beginning, a middle, and an end.

Titles

Powerful titles ensure attendance and attention at the opening of the session and are an important part of the introductory section. Below are some examples you could adapt for your own sessions.

Powerful titles (based on Kushner, 1997)

1 Use an exciting verb—*The Astonishing Role of the Macrophage.*

2 Adapt a song title/book title/movie title—*I want my, I want my, I want my ECG—Evidence-Based Practice in Ischaemic Heart Disease.*

3 Use a 'How to'—*How to make PowerPoint work for You.*

4 Use an analogy/saying—*There's many a slip twixt cup and lip—From Evidence to Practice.*

5 Use a number or ABC of—*Twelve Tips for the Successful Distance Learner.*

Introduction

This prepares the audience to listen and also prepares you to focus on your session. Make sure you grab the audiences' attention at the start. You have on average two minutes to get the interest of the audience and tell them what they are going to get out of the session before they decide whether they will switch off. Remember that a lot of what you put across is to do with *how* you say it and the non-verbal cues you give. Surprisingly little is to do with *what* you have to say. In your introduction walk confidently to podium and with a confident air present the opening of the lecture without notes. Keep the introduction simple and precise. Introduce yourself briefly and state why you have been asked to give the lecture if appropriate. An effective way of getting the audience on board is to personalize the experience. Make the session relevant to them or give a short personal anecdote to encourage them to relate to you as a person. Do not start with an apology about your lack of expertise or lack of preparation, it sets the wrong tone completely. Once you have introduced yourself and the topic, you should let the audience know what you intend to cover (the objectives).

Body

This is the main part of the presentation. Some of the key issues to think about in the body when talking to a large group are discussed below.

Clarity

This includes both your voice and the order in which you present material. You may need to speak at a rate that sounds fractionally slow to you and use more emphasis than sounds natural to your ear. Exhibit your enthusiasm through hand and facial gestures, and avoid jargon wherever possible.

Structure

There are two key ways to order the content of your lecture. If you are presenting the first in a series of lectures or introducing a new topic, it will help students to give them an overview of the subject. In other cases it will help them learn if you start from a specific example (see Chapter 5). Remember to break the content down into bite-sized chunks to accommodate the limitations of short-term memory. If the content is complex you will need to use some of the explaining skills outlined in Chapter 4. Use very explicit signposting and summarize as you move from one point to another, e.g. '*So we have covered the main points of the pathology of this condition and now we will move on to the ways in which the condition may present. . . .*'

At some point you may lose your place or your train of thought. If this happens try not to communicate your sense of panic. Pause, evaluate your situation, decide on a course of action, and continue. Often this may not even be noticed. If you are truly lost ask one of the audience to summarize what has been covered so far.

Presenting data

Verbal delivery of information can be unstimulating and so try to incorporate some audio-visual materials. However, data must be presented in a digestible and understandable form. Never find yourself saying '*Apologies for the busy slide . . .* '. Be careful in your choice of aids; they should complement not distract from your talk. If you do use audio-visual aids however, there will always be a time when things go wrong and so it is important to have back-up equipment or resources if possible. At least have some notes of what the slides or acetates contained to help you continue. Try not to get involved in the technical side of repairing the problem unless you know exactly what is wrong and how to fix it. If the repair work is prolonged, you may have to continue without your AV aids. Do not be tempted to pass material such as slides around, it will be irrelevant and distracting by the time most of the audience get to see it.

Questions

Ensure you have included enough time for questions and thought beforehand of the questions you would expect. Listen to each question carefully; if it is inaudible or complex restate it clearly. Be precise with your answers; sometimes yes or no is enough.

Close

As always you need to ensure that no new material is introduced here. Many lecturers end with the phrase '*Any questions?*' but this loses the presenter the opportunity to provide a powerful close with key take home messages. Remember that the audience often remembers the last things that were said and so it is a shame if this is an irrelevant point raised in an obscure question.

Interacting with a large group audience

Many lecturers will say that trying to introduce interaction into a large group session is unnecessary as well as unfeasible. In some cases they may be right. If you are presenting information only and expect students to follow this up with independent study then an entirely passive delivery may be OK for a very short lecture. If you want to go on for a longer period or want learning to happen at the time of the lecture you will need to let the audience interact with the material. This may be simply including questions but there are a number of other ways of introducing interaction in a large group setting. The most simple is to allow a couple of minutes regularly throughout the session for students to reflect on their notes taken so far. In this way students are benefiting from revision and a change in stimulus which may help student to retain both what you have already covered and to prepare for what you are about to cover. Getting students to work or interact with the material either by discussion in pairs or by asking questions also helps with encouraging active learning.

Ice-breakers

These are designed to simply get the group used to talking. If you wish the session to be interactive it is a good idea to get the first interactive episode in early to set the scene and allow the audience to know what is expected of them. Make the early exercises easy, e.g. simple introductions or comparing existing knowledge about the subject.

Pair work

Getting the audience to talk to the person next to them about some part of the session is possible in even the most steeply banked lecture theatre. Ensure there is a reason for the pair to talk. Give a specific task and a specific time frame in which to do it. For example, '*The last statement I made was rather a broad generalization and may not always be applicable to you. I would like you to turn to the person next to you and for the next two minutes first discuss to what extent each of you agree with the statement, and secondly give each other one or two examples in your experience where this generalization was difficult to apply*'.

Snowballing/buzz groups

This is an extension on pair work and involves pairs coming together with other pairs to share the discussion they have had in a pair. For example, '*I would now like you to turn to the pair behind you and for the next five minutes first see to what extent you all agree, and then list the reasons why there is disagreement. At the end of the time I will ask a spokesperson for each of the groups to describe the key features of what has been discussed*'.

This encourages further sharing of information and interaction with the material; it can help with reaching consensus and allows a spokesperson for the group if called upon to speak on behalf of a fair number of the audience rather than just himself. The pairs can keep joining with other groups until you have a manageable number of groups to get some views from all the groups in the room. In a banked lecture theatre with fixed seats the upper limit of a group is about eight but if you can move chairs you may be able to get larger groups.

Getting volunteers to answer or interact

Asking for a volunteer to participate or answer questions is a useful technique and is far better than picking on someone at random. However don't be fooled into checking the learning of the whole group from the responses of a volunteer. The larger the audience the more likely that this individual is not representative of the group. The best way to get volunteers is to prepare them for this task. Explain early on in the session that you be asking for comments from the group and that you will be asking questions. Better still, while the first few students are sauntering in engage them in conversation and then ask them if it would be OK to ask them to volunteer later in the session. Give them an idea of what you will be expecting and be sure to thank them for their contribution.

Quizzes

These can be useful at the beginning of the session, towards the end, or both. Having them at the beginning engages the audience, gets them thinking about the subject area, and can test and reactivate prior knowledge. Used both at the beginning and end or just at the end of a session they help to emphasize key points, check learning, and provide a sense of achievement. The quizzes do not need to be complex. They can be a show of hands, true false statements, MCQs, or completing statements. They should be self-marked but the results or answers can be shared with neighbours to identify common errors and reinforce the learning points.

Brainstorming

This can be difficult in a very large group but not impossible. You can modify the process for larger groups by using 'Post-it' notes or something similar and asking everyone to write down one idea. You will need some time to do some preliminary sorting into themes before writing the main themes onto the board. You could do this just before a break in a session. Alternatively buzz groups could be formed to process and theme the emerging material.

Questions

This is the commonest way of introducing interaction into a session. As with all interactions if you actually want the students to ask or answer questions set the scene early on. When asking questions try to use techniques that make more than one person come up with the answer such as getting everyone to write the answer down and asking for selected volunteers to share what they have written. Try to encourage students to ask you questions and to ask each other questions. In some situations you may want to limit the type and amount of questions asked. Be clear about this or else you may impede all questions. For example you might say '*There will be plenty of time for questions in this session but during this first section can we limit the questions to those about clarification please*'.

Many teachers are reluctant to encourage the audience to ask questions. They are worried they may be asked difficult questions to which they don't know the answer, or ones that are irrelevant and distracting. They also worry about hostile questions where the questioner has an ulterior motive. While these things do happen from time to time they are infrequent and not a good reason to leave questions out altogether. A really determined question asker will just interrupt and ask questions anyway. There are a few useful things you can do and think about that can prepare you for these uncomfortable but infrequent situations.

Difficult questions

Anticipate likely questions at the planning stage and prepare replies. If a question is difficult listen carefully to it, and then restate or paraphrase it. This will allow the whole audience to hear, and give you valuable thinking time. If you don't know the answer say so and consider asking the audience if they can answer it for you. This will almost certainly generate the answer (usually from the questioner) and will get the audience on your side.

Irrelevant questions

Be polite but try not to be drawn. Try saying '*That is a very interesting question and one I would be happy to discuss with you afterwards but perhaps now we can stick with the main points of the session*'.

Hostile questions

Try not to become defensive or angry. It is worth taking a step back and thinking about what the questioner is trying to achieve. It is usually not personal and is about attention seeking. Keep the questioner and audience on your side by being polite and precise. A long and convoluted statement masquerading as a question is sensibly answered with a simple 'yes' or 'no'. Reflecting back to the questioner your thoughts can also be powerful: '*You seem to want me to answer this question in a particular way. Why is that?*' This sort of questioner often wants to ask multiple questions often going over and over the same themes that they have particular views about. Don't get drawn into a game of 'question tennis'. Thank the questioner and suggest there may be others in the room who also want to ask some questions and move on. Usually if the atmosphere has become uncomfortable a kindly soul can be relied upon to ask a kinder question.

Large group teaching checklist

There is a lot to remember about a large group teaching session but when such sessions go well you normally have an enormous sense of achievement. It is worth developing or using a checklist to help you check your preparation for the session and to enable it to run effectively.

Large group teaching checklist

Introduction

- How will I establish an appropriate mood/get audience on board?
- Have I outlined utility/relevance to motivate students to learn?
- Have I described the content of the session?
- How will I establish or reactivate the knowledge base of students?
- Have I established what is expected of the audience?
- Have I planned to share objectives at the beginning of the session?
- Are the objectives clear/precise?

Summary

The number of students you are teaching is a key factor in deciding the objectives you might be able to achieve, the teaching methods you will use, and how you might check whether learning has happened. One to one teaching, small group teaching, and lecturing to large groups all have specific advantages and utilize a wide variety of skills. However, the main concepts that underpin effective teaching and learning; planning, structure, clarity of objectives, and active participation are all important whether you are teaching one or one hundred students.

(contd)

Body

1 Have I included techniques that make all the students come up with a response, e.g. all write their answer down.
2 Have I varied the stimulus?
3 Have I planned to emphasize major points?
4 Have I included enough interaction/active learning/time for questions?
5 How will I maintain interest?
6 Have I limited the amount of content?
7 Have I marked out sections that could be left out if time runs out?
8 When will I give out handouts?
9 Have I produced suitable AV aids?

Close

1 Have I planned to summarize key points?

References

Belbin, R. M. (1981) *Management teams—why they succeed or fail.* Butterworth Heinmann.

Brown, G., and Manogue, M. (2001) AMEE Medical Education Guide No. 22: Refreshing lecturing: a guide for lecturers. **23**, 231–44.

Cox, K. (1993) Planning bedside teaching. *Med J Aust* **158**, 280–2.

Crosby, J. (1997) *AMEE educational guide No. 8. Learning in small groups.* Dundee: AMEE.

Gibbs, G., and Habeshaw, T. (ed.) (1989) *Preparing for teaching TES publications.* Bristol: TES Publications.

Heron, J. (1989) Dimensions of facilitator style. In *Preparing for teaching TES publications* (ed. G. Gibbs and T. Habeshaw) Bristol: TES Publications.

Kushner, M. (1997) *Successful presentations for dummies.* California: IDG Books Worldwide Inc.

Race, P., and Brown, G. (1998) *The lecturer's toolkit.* London: Kogan Page.

Tuckman, B. (1965) Developmental sequence in small groups. *Psychol Bull* **LXIII**.

Further reading

Brown, G., and Manogue, M. (2001) AMEE Medical Education Guide No. 22: Refreshing lecturing: a guide for lecturers. **23**, 231–44.

Jaques, D. (1991) *Learning in groups.* London: Kogan Page.

Newble, D. and Cannon, R. (1994) *A handbook for medical teachers,* 3rd edn. London: Kluwer Academic Publishers.

CHAPTER 8

Teaching in the clinical setting

Introduction

Armed with your lesson plan and toolkit of teaching skills, delivering your teaching session should not seem too daunting. There are a multitude of potential settings in which you can deliver your teaching, from a lecture hall to a domiciliary visit. All these teaching settings can be divided into two key types: those in the '**service setting**' where you carry on with your clinical work simultaneously and those where you have '**protected time**' with your students. Teaching in protected time means that your clinical responsibilities are covered by another clinician, allowing you to teach without interruption. In practice, the majority of our medical teaching is done in the service setting. Bearing in mind our service commitments as well as the needs of the students, the patient, the medical school, the trust, and ourselves, is a difficult balancing act.

Must check his scan results and see his relatives
Probably tension like mine!
I'll come and catheterize Mr Yu in 10 minutes, just let me finish teaching
So, students, what do you think might be the cause of Mrs Brown's headaches?
Beep Beep!

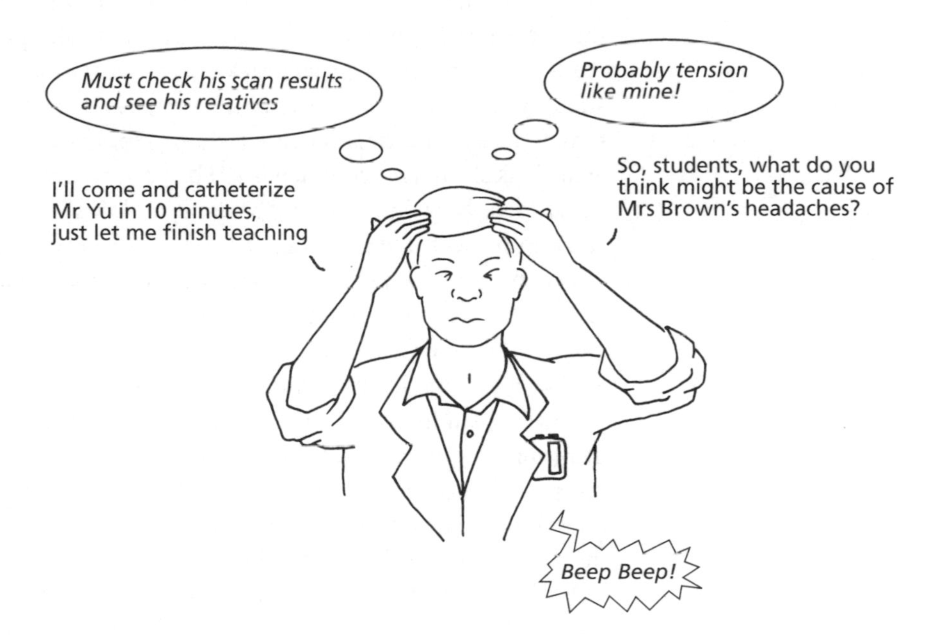

Teaching in protected time is usual in lectures and seminars and is often used to teach clinical and communication skills. It may also be used in bedside teaching, using patients who have been specifically selected for teaching. Teaching in the service setting covers any type of teaching that accompanies clinical work. This chapter looks at teaching in a variety of different clinical settings and suggests how the clinician can make optimum use of these settings to teach students effectively.

Doctors traditionally learned their craft in an apprenticeship model where new doctors observed their experienced colleagues at work. If they were lucky there was a structured progression from observing, through understanding, to acting as a doctor, in a graded series of logical steps. If they were unlucky then they might have been asked to do tasks for which they were unprepared and to perform these tasks unsupported. They also ran the risk of not covering the content of the medical curriculum. Because of these problems, there is a trend for medical schools to move towards a more structured way of providing clinical experience. Postgraduate training schemes, run by the Royal Colleges are now well organized along lines that produce confident safe doctors. However there is not yet a similar universal scheme for clinical undergraduates although there are many instances of good practice in different medical schools.

Until recently the vast majority of student learning took place on the wards. Changes in service provision have meant that patients are only admitted if they are acutely ill and discharged rapidly to follow-up care in the community. As a result there are fewer patients in hospital and many are too ill for students to clerk. To increase students exposure to clinical material, many schools have started to develop teaching in outpatients and primary care (referred to in the United States as '**ambulatory care**'). This gives valuable exposure to clinical cases (Malley *et al.*, 1999), but has some limitations. It may offer a narrow range of clinical material, can be unpredictable, may lack continuity, and be of variable quality. Students are said to examine patients rarely and have little time to discuss a case or receive feedback from teachers (Irby, 1995).

The added value of clinical teaching

Given that teaching in the clinical setting is difficult, why do we do it? Perhaps the most important reason is that it automatically places all the learning done by students in context. This will make the information easier to recall when a similar situation is encountered. Secondly, it prepares students for the sort of work they will have to face as clinicians. Finally, it shows them how a clinician uses their clinical and generic skills in their clinical work. The performance of the clinician is used to show the student how things should be done, and this is called '**role modelling**'. When we teach in protected time we can show students how we approach patients, clinical, or ethical problems, using interaction with real or simulated patients, case discussions, and problem solving exercises. However our actual performance in outpatients, surgery, or on the wards is likely to be a more powerful influence. This ability to provide a clinical role model distinguishes the clinical from the non-clinical teacher.

Medical students will automatically observe the way we treat patients as well as our interactions with non-medical colleagues and other staff such as ward clerks or receptionists. They will see how we cope with telephone calls during a clinic, with a tearful patient, or angry relative. They may watch us examining patients, carrying out clinical procedures, or breaking bad news. Demonstrating our own professional behaviour and attitudes and at the same time analysing and discussing them is a powerful way to set students along the path to becoming a professional. Role modelling takes place whether we refer to it overtly or not, and when we teach in the clinical setting we have the responsibility of acting as a positive role model.

Being an effective clinical teacher

Medicine is a practical subject and it is vital that students learn to be effective hands-on clinicians. To do this they need to work with their basic science knowledge and skills in the clinical setting. Currently much clinical teaching involves students as passive observers, to the detriment of their learning. Effective clinical teachers provide stimulating interactive experience for their students using the toolkit described in Chapter 4. If you are teaching in the service setting you need to call on some extra organizational skills to help you teach while you work.

Teaching with patients

Teaching in the clinical setting has the advantage of using real patients. This raises the challenge for students, but requires close supervision by teachers to ensure that the patients are comfortable. Students can learn more from some patients than others. Patients for teaching should be friendly, available, and willing to talk or be examined by students at the appropriate time. They often feel that teaching students is a way of making sense of their illness or learning more about it.

Patients that will help the students learn may have a good story to tell the students (this may be about their experiences of illness/health care and need not be limited to just an interesting medical history), or have good, ideally stable, clinical signs. There should be no significant communication barriers, unless you are teaching specifically about how to deal with communication difficulties. Sometimes teaching with a patient may help his/her medical care; for example, if you want to have a full detailed history taken and recorded in the notes, or consider an aspect of care that you have not previously explored.

Patients are usually very happy to take part in teaching sessions but it is wise to obtain permission explicitly and record that you have done so. Think about providing written as well as oral information when asking a patient's consent. You could create a specific information sheet about the teaching to give to patients when you are recruiting/consenting them to participate, or use the one below, which is designed for bedside teaching.

Teaching medical students

A guide for patients

Thank you for your interest in teaching our medical students. This sheet tells you what to expect from the session.

- The aim of the session will be to ____
- There will be __________ students from year _________ of the medical course.
- The students will want to talk to you and/or examine you.
- If you don't want to answer a question, just say "I would rather not answer that".
- If you feel unwell or uncomfortable with the teaching tell the teacher who will stop the session. This will in no way affect your medical care.
- Students may suggest some unlikely causes for your symptoms. If you have any concerns about what you hear, please talk with the teacher after the session.
- Medical students are bound by the same rules of confidentiality as doctors and will not disclose anything they have heard with anyone apart from your medical team.
- Tell your teacher after the session if you have any concerns about any of the students.

Consent to teaching

I ____ am happy to help teaching medical students, and understand that they wish to talk to me and/or examine me.

Date

Before any teaching session that involves patients it is important to prepare the patient, yourself, and the students. Think about covering the following:

Preparing for teaching with patients

Brief the patient

- The aim of the teaching session (e.g. to practise talking to patients).
- Any special instructions ("Don't tell them your diagnosis").
- Students numbers, and the level they are at.
- What the students will do, and for how long.
- The sort of questions students will ask (they do not have to answer them all).
- How to stop the teaching at any time.
- That students are bound by the same rules of medical confidentiality as doctors.
- Remind them that inexperienced students can suggest some unlikely diagnoses.

Brief yourself

- Check the clinical findings.
- Check the students have not seen the patient before.
- Check the students learning objectives—will this experience help their learning?

Brief the students

- Give ground rules for session (e.g. what to discuss or not in front of the patient).
- Discuss learning objectives.
- Discuss structure and allocate roles.

Teachers and fellow students are not the only ones who can give useful feedback on students' performance. Your patients can also be very helpful and insightful. Asking a patient to compare the examination skills of an experienced clinician with a medical student can be revealing and useful, showing the student how much pressure to use in an abdominal examination for example. Do not forget the patient's presence—it can be easy to get carried away with questioning and discussion while the patient may be worrying about the implications for him/her of your discussion.

Using your basic organizational and teaching skills

All of the skills covered in Chapter 4 are vital in the clinical setting. Just as in a non-clinical setting you will need to be organized, prepare the content, structure the session, and apply your basic teaching skills.

Prepare the clinical teaching session

Plan what you are going to teach, prepare the patient, and collect together useful clinical resources before the students arrive.

Structure the clinical teaching session

Maintain a clear introduction, body, and close to your session to help students learn. Pay particular attention to the introduction: establishing relevance and prior knowledge is vital, as is negotiating the objectives of the session with the students. Plan as much hands-on experience as possible and allow time for reflection at the close of the session.

Use your generic teaching skills

Particularly important in the clinical setting are getting the learning environment right, giving concise and logical explanations, using questions that explore higher levels of knowledge, and giving specific and constructive feedback. Break clinical skills teaching into small manageable chunks. Give clear demonstrations and ensure students understand **why** as well as **how** the skill is performed. Offer all students hands-on practice and encourage repeated practice on other patients.

Teaching in the clinical setting is often a little more complicated than this however. To make the most of the time you have with the students it helps to pay particular attention to the structure of the body of your session, promoting learning through active experience followed by reflection, integration of basic sciences, and the learning environment.

Much of the literature on clinical teaching comes from America. Research has shown that clinical teachers often spend little time teaching at the bedside. 50% of clinical teaching time is spent in seminar rooms, 25% at the bedside, and students get to demonstrate their clinical skills for less than 5% of the time. Clinical teachers often have little idea about their students learning needs, and tend to focus on knowledge objectives which could be met by other means. The lack, in many schools, of a method of communicating students progress to teachers, often leads to teaching that is inappropriately pitched. Clinical teachers often lack a clear idea of the overall curriculum, which in any case is often insufficiently detailed to guide them (Cox, 1993).

Encouraging teachers to make the most of each teaching session means increasing the amount of relevant 'hands-on' experience, and using a model that maximizes learning from each patient encounter. Harth *et al.* (1992) studied clinical learning environments in Australia, and found many suboptimal learning environments, considerable criticism of tutors with less than half being considered effective teachers, and disturbing reports from a third of students of mistreatment by their tutors.

Using clinical teaching skills

We often call teaching with patients 'bedside teaching' although many patients are mobile. Even in protected time, teaching with a patient is more complicated than other teaching as your attention must be split between the students and the patient.

Students will learn most effectively when they are involved with their learning, and the key to learning in the clinical setting is encouraging contact with the patient and involvement in their care.

Structuring the session

Learning in the clinical setting is based on experience, and we know that experiential learning requires not only an experience, but also time to reflect on that experience (see Chapter 2). The experiential learning model has been redrawn for clinical teachers by Cox, and is a useful way to structure the body of your clinical session.

The clinical teaching model shows two main cycles: an experience and an explanation cycle. Within the experience cycle you first '**brief**' your students about the patient they are going to see. This briefing acts as an advance organizer, creating the framework into which the new information can be fitted. The clinical experience needs to be as 'hands-on' as possible: it will not be possible for all your students to take a full history, but you should be able to ensure that they all take some part in the activity. After the clinical experience, your students need to be '**debriefed**' to ensure that they saw and understood everything that they experienced.

Many teachers stop at this point, missing a golden opportunity for reinforcing student learning by moving on into the '**explanation cycle**'. Within this, you get students to reflect on their experiences by asking 'What did that mean'. This allows them to connect the experience to previous experiences and to develop deeper meanings. From this they can develop explanations of 'What went on' drawing together information from their knowledge of clinical medicine and the basic sciences. To develop their working knowledge, think about asking your students '*What would you do next time?*' and get them to think about what further learning they may need to do to help them.

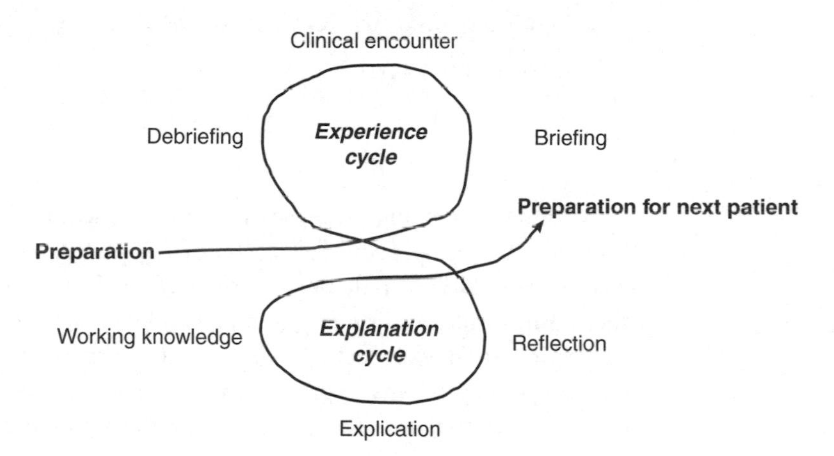

Figure 8.1 A model for clinical teaching (Cox 1993)

The cycle shows clearly how students experience can be converted into useful working knowledge. Teaching a skill requires specialized approaches that form part of the experience cycle and are addressed in Chapter 5. In the clinical setting, the two skills which cause the most difficulties for students are the commonest two of the clinical activities: performing a medical interview and clinical reasoning.

Teaching clinical reasoning

All medical students find making diagnoses difficult. They are not helped by the fact that they will see you making diagnoses in two distinct ways: pattern recognition in easy cases and hypothesis testing in difficult ones (see Chapter 5). As pattern recognition requires considerable clinical experience, students start off using hypothesis testing.

Making useful hypotheses is only possible if students are in the right 'ball park', and you can get them there more quickly by encouraging them to think carefully about the key features of a patient's problem. This means getting them to stop, think, and commit to a 'ball park' (e.g. "This problem is chest pain") early on in the interview, and to then test out the idea within the interview. Once they have committed themselves to a ball park, you then need to ask them to:

(a) **Reflect**—and consider what ideas come to mind when 'hearing' the early representation or key features.

(b) **Plan**—what further questions or examination would help them establish a diagnoses?

(c) **Experiment**—proceed with further questions and examination.

The process of teaching clinical reasoning has been summarized for use in the clinical setting by Neher *et al.* (1992) using the system below known as 'The One Minute Preceptor', which is said to add only a minute to average teaching time.

Enhancing clinical reasoning at the bedside

1 Commitment (ask the student to state what he thinks is going on).

2 Probe for supporting evidence (why do you think this?).

3 Teach general rules.

4 Reinforce correct assumptions of good ideas with positive feedback.

5 Correct mistakes.

We don't make things easier for students by encouraging them to present detailed histories in a pre-set fashion. This 'reporter' approach interferes with the 'detective' approach that will help them get to the right ball park, produce hypotheses, and test them out. Instead of listening to a classical presentation, try asking students what they think are the key features and why they are important. This is more likely to encourage the students to process the information they are gathering. We can also encourage detective behaviour by using the following framework when getting students to present their findings:

Enhancing clinical reasoning in case presentations

Focus	Ask the student to focus their findings into a brief summary.
Wait	Wait for them to finish describing what they feel are the key findings. Hold your tongue! Don't ask factual recall questions.
What?	Ask the student what they think the diagnosis or management plan is.
Why?	Ask them to justify their reasoning. What led them to these conclusions?
Uncertainty	Ask them what they are uncertain about. Do any features make them uncertain?
Give feedback	Reinforce what they did well and explain where they could have done better.

We can also use other techniques to improve clinical reasoning skills:

- Let them know how *you* do it. Try thinking out loud; talk through your decisions, how you weigh the evidence, and what influences your choices.

- Voice your uncertainty. We rarely allow students to realize that there are clear limits to our own knowledge and skill, because we think (unfairly) that they will think less of us. It would help students voice their uncertainties if we were explicit about our own. Admit if you are making decisions merely on a hunch, because of a past missed diagnosis or because you are unsure what to do next.

- Choose a common condition to teach clinical reasoning. Try to ensure that the students have some useful clinical knowledge relevant to the case so they can concentrate on making decisions, and ensure that the mood of the session is safe and non-judgemental.

- Improve pattern recognition skills by encouraging your students to see common conditions repeatedly. Teaching by comparison between cases rather than teaching each condition separately improves pattern recognition.

In difficult cases clinicians rely on both their clinical knowledge and their underlying knowledge of the basic sciences to solves cases. With the increasing integration of medical courses, teaching the basic sciences is no longer the remit of anatomists and pathologists and clinical teachers can help students by integrating their basic medical science understanding into their teaching.

Integrating the basic sciences

We want students to understand the basic science underlying clinical medicine so that they can solve the clinical problems they will face in the future. Early medical educators (Flexner, 1910) thought that by exposing students to courses in the basic sciences, they would be automatically able to call upon this knowledge when needed. You may remember from your own medical school experience that this approach was not always effective. Most medical schools now have an integrated curriculum where students learn anatomy, physiology, biochemistry, and pathology of systems in parallel. The final piece of the learning jigsaw is for this learning to be placed in the clinical context. It is tempting to assume that if your students learned in an integrated curriculum, they won't need help with integrating knowledge. However the clinical setting can be so overwhelming, that it is sometimes difficult for students to identify useful knowledge that can help them.

The way in which you address integrating the basic sciences and problem solving depends on the setting. In protected time, you might start by revising the underlying anatomy and physiology of the topic. The aim of this is twofold—first to integrate the relevant sciences, but also to allow students to identify the foundation onto which they will add the new information. You may then be able to go through the problem solving process with the students in detail. In the service setting, you are likely to have less time to teach the students, and making the most of the limited time you have at your disposal is vital. In this case role modelling becomes more important. It may be possible to talk through what you are doing, or use Cox's technique of 'brief–debrief–reflect' at the beginning and end of the experience to succinctly explore relevant information.

'One of the pleasures of teaching clinical students in their early encounters with patients is to see the sudden moments of delight as they realize that the hard learned anatomy of the cranial nerves makes sense when they see a patient with a cranial nerve palsy'.

Getting the pitch and pace right

Getting the pitch and pace of a teaching session right is important, and there is no substitute for spending time with the students defining their learning objectives, assessing their prior knowledge, confidence and competence in skills, and negotiating what you are going to teach. If you are short of time in the clinical setting it is tempting to leave this out. Given that this is likely to lead to unsuccessful teaching sessions, an alternative solution is to use the short time that you have efficiently. If you are a regular clinical teacher (for example a firm leader), it may be possible to meet with the students at the start of the attachment and spend a session talking through what they hope to achieve during the time that they are with you. Using the list they generate (and your knowledge of the actual aims and objectives of the attachment) you may be able to negotiate a series of teaching sessions, which could take place on ward rounds, in clinic, or in theatre. Because you have already defined their prior knowledge and agreed the objectives of the session, once you find yourself with an appropriate patient and a little time you can start immediately.

As an occasional teacher you will have more problems. If the students have already spent time with their main teacher defining what they want to learn, they may be able to tell you quite precisely what they plan to cover. If this is not the case, then it is wise to spend as much time as you can on setting the session up, and then continually check with the students that you are getting the level right. Students may not want to upset you and say that the session meets their needs, but by monitoring their body language, you may get a clear idea of their actual opinions.

And the possible causes of death in this syndrome are...?
Boredom?

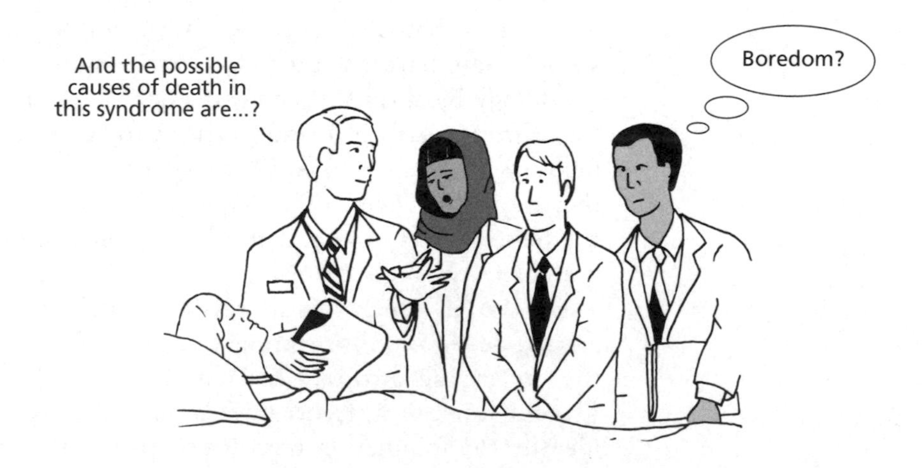

Finding out what your students know before you start every session may seem rather repetitive. If you teach in a specialist field, it is likely that when you ask your students '*What do you know about dermatitis herpetiformis*' their knowledge will be limited. However don't try to guess what they do and don't know, unless you know both the students and the session well. Even an experienced teacher is likely to get it wrong. Tutors in specialist fields may quickly find out what students know about the area, while tutors in more generic areas of medicine and surgery will need to spend more time establishing the limits of their students' knowledge, confidence, and competence. Transmitting what you know about a student's or group of students' knowledge to other teachers is very useful, but can be difficult in practice unless you document what you have discovered.

Using logbooks

Not only may tutors have difficulty finding out what students know, but students often worry about what they should be learning on clinical attachments, because course guides are either too vague or too detailed. Medical schools have tried out several ways of communicating the curriculum and recording students ongoing achievements in a portable form, and many are currently using paper-based logbooks. These show the student what is expected of them and can be used to check what they have actually achieved.

Sample page from a logbook

These procedures can be performed and observed in the clinical skills laboratory and theatre.

Perform	Practice 1	Practice 2	Practice 3	Competent
Surgical scrub procedure				
Inserting IV cannula				
Bag-mask ventilation				
Oral/nasal airway insertion				
Airway management				
Demonstrate CPR–manikin				
Insert a urinary catheter				
Use 3-lead ECG monitor				
Suture skin				

Observe	Seen date 1	Seen date 2	Seen date 3
Arterial blood gas sampling			
Radial arterial cannulation			
Blood transfusion			
Insertion of a CVP line			
Tracheal intubation			
Arterial and CVP monitoring			
Artificial ventilation			
Giving IV fluids			

However while logbooks are a useful aid memoire they do have disadvantages. Ideally a logbook will identify pre-set and negotiated learning objectives, will document the existing strengths and weaknesses of the student in the area, will contain checklists for essential competencies, and include an area for additional or more generic activities and achievements to be documented. However logbooks are often little more than a set of fixed objectives and a skills checklist.

Another problem is that logs cannot reflect the reiterative process involved in learning clinical skills and applying them to subsequent clinical situations. For example you might 'sign off' a student as competent in examining the heart. This will reflect examination of the heart once in one particular setting. The tick does not indicate the level of skill the student has achieved, i.e. if he/she is sufficiently competent to examine the heart in an obese patient, or one with different pathology. There is no indication whether the student understands the underlying principles of using a stethoscope or of production of heart murmurs.

Another disadvantage is that logbooks are a good example of assessment driving learning: if logs are regularly assessed by teachers, students may be keen only to 'get signed up' rather than make the most of teaching episodes. If teachers neglect the logs, then so will the students.

To be useful, and to motivate students to use them, logbooks need to be reviewed during a course as well as at the end. This checks that progress is occurring and helps the teacher and student to plan activities in the remaining time. It can also be useful for determining how unmet needs might be addressed.

To observe a student's performance, give feedback, and sign him/her as competent takes time and a quiet place to talk. Unfortunately teachers are often approached by students at inconvenient moments on ward rounds or in drafty corridors.

Getting the environment right

While seminar rooms and lecture theatres have been designed for teaching, wards, consulting rooms, and theatres are not. Getting the physical and psychological environment right is very important for learning. In the clinical setting, this can vary from simple measures such as making sure that there are enough chairs, to preparing students to see particular patients or clinical problems. On the wards, moving out of a busy corridor into a side room for a swift opportunistic teaching encounter allows everyone to concentrate on the teaching session. In the clinic or general practice setting, careful arrangement of the room can include the undergraduate as a learner, can encourage active rather than passive participation, and can provide support for the undergraduate in an unfamiliar setting. Think about placing the students where they can have eye contact with you and the patient. Try not to put your students behind the patient or you may find they quickly adopt a passive role. The desk can also act as a barrier.

Summary

The essence of being an effective clinical teacher has been summarized by Newble and Cannon (1994) in eight key points which are worth bearing in mind before you start any clinical teaching session.

Eight attributes of an effective clinical teacher

1. Encourages active rather than passive observation.
2. Concentrates on teaching of applied problem solving.
3. Integrates clinical medicine with basic science.
4. Observes students closely during interview/examination rather than during side room case presentation.
5. Provides adequate opportunity for students to practise skills.
6. Provides a good role model for interpersonal relationships with patients.
7. Teaches in a patient orientated rather than disease orientated fashion.
8. Demonstrates a positive attitude towards teaching.

Teaching in the service setting

Teaching while trying to care for your patients can be particularly stressful. Bleeps, phone calls, colleagues, and patients may interrupt the session and put you and your students under considerable strain. A common way to cope with this is to force the student into a passive role 'sitting in with Nelly' and hope that he/she will just pick something up as you go along. This is not an effective way for a student to learn. He/she needs to be involved in the clinical session and learning in an active manner.

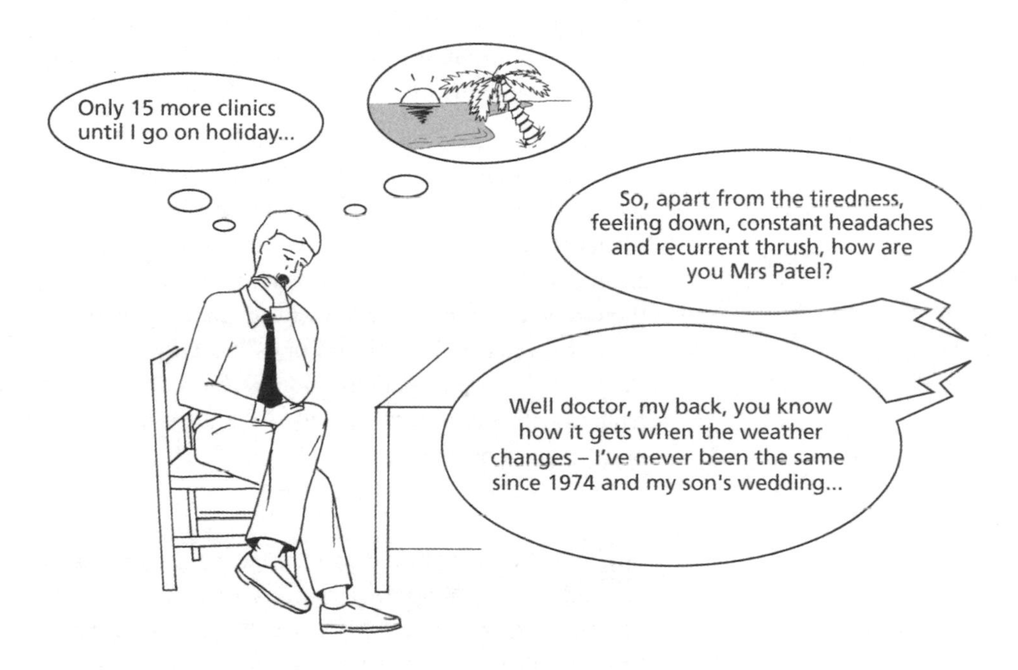

When teaching in clinic, on the wards, or in practice, it is worthwhile trying to minimize disruption whilst maximizing the opportunities for learning. This means thinking about organizational issues as well as choosing a structure for your teaching.

Organizational issues

Addressing the organization of your clinical work will permit you more flexibility and more time to teach. How you organize your teaching will depend on where the teaching is going on, the number of rooms and staff available, and the number of students. We will deal with specific techniques under the different settings.

Structuring teaching

Reorganizing your clinical load will buy you some time, but not enough to deliver a lengthy teaching session. To teach efficiently you will need to modify your teaching methods. Cox's model of clinical teaching with its dual cycles of preparation/brief/experience/debrief/reflect can be used in the service setting but can take a lot of time if you use it with every experience. Several other effective techniques can be used that utilize some aspect of the cycle. The methods you use will depend on the setting, the time you have available, and when in the clinical episode the teaching segment arises.

- *All action.* Continue with your activity but fit in a three minute 'round up' regularly. During this you and the learner should summarize what you have seen and learned.
- *Planning–action.* This equates to just using the 'experience cycle', and is useful if you have some time at the start of the session to explore prior knowledge and set objectives before the list or clinic begins.
- *Action–reflection.* This equates to using just the 'reflection cycle'. If you are pressed this will have to take place at the end of the clinical session, but it is helpful to do several times during the session.
- *Trigger.* This involves negotiating beforehand what you will teach about—thus when an appropriate patient or opportunity arrives you can begin the teaching segment.

In general it helps to brief students by telling them what to expect. Explain that you are establishing at the beginning what the student hopes to gain from time with you so you can focus your teaching accordingly. Keep interest and motivation up by involving students in patient care as much as possible. This can range from performing small clinical tasks—taking blood pressure—to fully clerking the patient and presenting them to you. In a busy clinical setting, this may require some lateral thinking: students could be asked to look things up—"*Could you check whether digoxin interacts with fluoxetine*", observe patients non-verbal communication, assist nurses to set up trolleys with equipment, or write case notes. The latter would need careful checking before you signed them.

Teachers find it problematic to juggle clinical and teaching loads (Skeff *et al.*, 1997). Experienced teachers, however seem to be able to combine learner centred approaches with sound educational practices, broad learning experiences, attention to student learning, and concern for development of professional expertise and judgement (Mann *et al.*, 2001). They do this by a combination of skilled teaching and organizational changes to their clinical commitments which permit them to maximize their time with the students (Usatine *et al.*, 2000).

Remember that 'less is more'. If you attempt in-depth teaching on every patient you will be stressed and run late. Finally, even in a busy clinic, try not to start without an introduction or miss closing the session—build on what students have learned before you let them go.

Teaching in specific service settings

Teaching on the wards

Teaching on the wards is usually highly rated by students. The special features of teaching at the bedside are the presence of the patient, availability of notes with all investigations, X-rays, drug and nursing charts, and teaching in a small group. Bedside teaching can be organized in several different ways, of which the most common are:

- Business rounds: students observe the 'real work' of the clinical team.
- Teaching rounds: these are set up specifically for teaching using patients selected by the teacher and often already seen by the students. While teaching ward rounds are theoretically held in protected time, in practice they are often interrupted by clinical work.

- Small group bedside teaching: these usually involve only one patient, and a small group of students, and are often used in clinical skills teaching.
- Patient centred model: students are allocated certain patients to follow during their admission.
- Shadowing: students follow a junior member of staff and share in their work as much as possible.

Centring student's teaching around patients is logical and, unless the firm is very large, it is also practical. Students should be encouraged to clerk patients when they are admitted (ideally in the Accident and Emergency department), follow them daily, and take the responsibility of presenting them to the team on ward rounds. Encouraging students to read around their cases will help to integrate the basic sciences. Remember that students may find presenting stressful so ensure you foster a climate where it is OK to make mistakes and express uncertainty. Asking students to present their clerking on business rounds slows the round down, so you might make it their responsibility to present only part of the history—for example the last day's progress, or latest blood results. If you expect students to attend business rounds, it may be helpful to give them a task to focus on during the round, e.g. communication with patients and staff or decision making. Alternatively you could suggest that your students only stay for the first half of the round, and then work towards some agreed learning objective for the second half. Make some time and space after the ward round to talk through what they have been doing.

On all ward rounds position the patient, student, and yourself so you can see everyone and gauge the extent of their engagement in the session.

Involving students as much as possible in talking about patient care is important. During ward-based teaching you will have the chance of observing and giving feedback to your students on their clinical skills. This is a vital time for learning. Make sure that any feedback given is immediate and constructive and if necessary find a place to do this away from the main ward round. Consider asking the patient and other students to give feedback to the student.

Teaching in outpatients

Outpatient teaching is beneficial for students as they can see large amounts of 'clinical material' in a short space of time. However it can be difficult for doctors trying to run a clinic and boring for students if they are watching passively. Some organizational changes will be easy to make—for example altering the position of chairs, while others—finding extra rooms, changing the scheduling of your clinic, or persuading colleagues to help you teach—will be more difficult.

Structuring your teaching in outpatients depends on the number of students you have to accommodate and the number of teachers available. If you have one or two students then the options are 'sitting in', using an apprenticeship model, or using a separate room for the students to see patients and then report back to you. The apprenticeship model involves the student conducting the medical interview with the doctor watching. While this is an excellent learning experience for the student it takes time. Allowing the students to see patients in another room relies on careful clinic scheduling, but will not take up extra time. If time and space are at a premium then 'sitting in' is your only option. To maximize learning, try to find some time before the session to discuss learning objectives and consider setting the students 'observer tasks', e.g.

'The next three patients are all new patients. I want you to make a differential diagnosis/list of appropriate tests/rate how patient centred I am being in the consultation, and then we will discuss your findings'.

Students with more experience may be able to write the clinic notes, draft clinic letters, or take part in small ways in the examination and management of the patient. While seeing a patient alone is very popular with students, it has the disadvantage that no one can observe and give useful feedback on their performance.

Larger groups of students present problems. Big groups in the clinic room are intimidating for patients, so it may be useful to use a 'boomerang' model where students go and do things and then report back. But, because students are seeing the patient alone, you will not know whether they have performed the task correctly. An alternative is the 'breakout' model, where the students first observe you at work and then repeat or expand on what you have been doing with patients on their own.

With really large groups of students, you can divide the students among the available tutors. Remember to include other health professionals such as dieticians and nurses. An alternative is to allocate all the students to one tutor whose clinical workload is then reduced so they can see specially selected patients. A final option is the 'shuttle' model, where the students wait in a central pool and are called in to see particularly interesting patients. To use these models successfully you will need to tell students and staff exactly what you plan to do.

Many models for teaching in ambulatory care have been developed. Eleven of these are reviewed by Heidenreich *et al.* (2000). It seems likely that following an initial orientation to the clinical setting (DaRosa *et al.*, 1997), students will benefit from an approach that structures the teaching experience, using learning objectives agreed by the tutor and the student. Agreeing learning objectives is easier if there is sufficient time, and the teacher and students have worked together before (Laidley *et al.*, 2000). Techniques that maximize the time available for teaching include scheduling appointments so that there are patients available for the student to examine, getting students to do their case presentations in the examination room (Ferenchick *et al.*, 1997), and asking the students to write the notes (Usatine *et al.*, 2000). This maximizes students involvement in patient care leading to improved learning.

Teaching in general practice

General practice teaching takes place in two main ways—teaching about general practice, often called 'core general practice teaching' which takes place in the service setting, and clinical skills teaching usually in protected time. General practice is the ideal setting to learn about consultation skills, and you may wish to teach about consultation skills as well as the clinical content of your work. Students are usually sent to practices alone or in small groups. This, along with the resources of the primary care team, can make organizing teaching easier than in a busy clinic. There are plenty of things for students to do, but it is worthwhile spending time with your students initially to tailor the available learning experiences to their needs.

Students in general practice commonly 'sit in' with their GP teacher. This is a useful way to experience the work that GPs do and see consultation skills in action. However, particularly in busy surgeries, it can be a very passive experience for the student. Try to ensure that students have a mix of surgeries and other activities during a day in your practice. You can involve the student in the surgery by:

- Giving them simple clinical tasks e.g. '*Would you mind taking Mrs Brown's blood pressure for me*'.
- Asking them to look thing up for you (drug interactions, blood results).
- Getting them to act as observers with a specific task to do (e.g. '*Observe how I summarize my findings during the consultation in the next three consultations*').
- Asking them to see patients initially in another room and present them to you.
- Asking them to occasionally interview the patient in your presence.

Try and spend time with your students at the beginning and end of each surgery to brief and debrief. You may find it helpful to reorganize your workload by putting in regular breaks (e.g. blocking off every fifth patient to give you a breathing space). Your partners are also a valuable resource: 'sitting in' with them and contrasting their consultation styles with your own may be a useful exercise for the student.

One potential disadvantage of 'core general practice teaching' is that it can be tiring to be responsible for one student continuously for two or three weeks. Planning breaks for yourself while students do projects, home visits, or work with partners or other members of the team can relieve the pressure.

Teaching on call in the Accident and Emergency Department

Students find the atmosphere of A+E motivating but can also be intimidated. They appreciate that clinical teachers are often very busy, and do not expect the same intensity of teaching that they might get in other clinical settings. However, A+E is an excellent learning environment for students, not only for clinical skills but also for generic skills.

The way in which you organize and structure teaching in A+E depends on the number of students and your clinical load. Possibly the best way is to have one or two students shadowing each clinician. If you are rushed off your feet or in an emergency situation, simply describing what you are doing out loud including explaining the decisions you are making is an effective way of teaching and including students.

If there is a large group of students a 24 hour period can be divided up between them, not forgetting that in many hospitals there are facilities for students to stay overnight. Use a quiet moment at the beginning of the attachment or day to establish the students' knowledge base and experience. Planning how to spend the hours together will be well worth the effort. With a small number of students it should be possible to give them some supervised involvement and responsibility (although not so much that they are overwhelmed). It is critical to be sure that a student is competent before asking them to perform a task. Make sure that they understand that they can refuse to do something if they are not confident enough. Let the student take a history and examine a patient before you do, ask him to present patients to you, and allow him to have first go at interpreting test results. At the end of the on call time go through the patients you have seen and discuss the useful learning points. Remember also that other medical and non-medical staff have much to contribute to medical student learning in this setting.

Teaching in theatre

This can be very interesting and exciting for students if they can see what is going on, if they have had a chance to brush up on their anatomy, physiology, and pathology, or if they know or have clerked the patient. Students like to feel useful and are very happy to assist in an operation even in the most minor capacity where they can feel a valued part of the team. Try to ensure all students present have an unobstructed view of the procedure. If this is not possible consider using different learning activities for different students and perhaps call on the other professionals present during the list to engage the students in other tasks.

Theatre is a place for students to learn about surgery and anaesthetics. Learning is maximized because it is in context. For the surgeon, there may be time before the list to talk to the students, while the anaesthetist may have opportunities while the patient is on the table. If at all possible students should have seen the patients on the list. It is useful to brief the students about what they will see, and think about how you can promote active learning rather then passive observation. With the development of minimally invasive surgery, there are fewer roles for students in theatres. With the use of monitors however, students may have a very good view of the operative field and can be prompted to review their anatomical knowledge as well as learning about surgery. Many anaesthetic techniques are taught best in skills laboratories, but it is also important for the students to observe them being carried out in context. Theatres may be the only place that students can practise on real patients in putting in IV lines and so time in the anaesthetic room is well spent. Of course you will make sure that patients have given consent for all procedures you may ask the students to perform.

In between patients and during gaps in lists, surgeons and anaesthetists could make good use of time by running *ad hoc* tutorials on one of the knowledge areas from the students list of objectives. To maximize this time negotiate with students beforehand which subject areas you are likely to discuss. Try to encourage dialogue rather than monologue and thus more active learning.

Teaching in protected time

Teaching in protected time often seems like a luxury after trying to teach in the service setting. Protected time allows you time to deliver a planned session, and an opportunity to observe students closely and offer feedback.

Some teaching in protected time takes place at the bedside: either on the wards or in general practice. Other teaching uses the specialized settings of the clinical skills centre and the consultation skills suite.

It is important that your time is truly protected as interruptions by telephone calls or bleeps will interfere with the smooth running of the teaching session, affect the quality of the students learning, and increase your stress levels.

Clinical skills centre

The clinical skills centre is the ideal place for medical students to practise their clinical skills. It offers a safe, controlled, and supervised environment. Equipment may range from very straightforward models of a breast for examination of lumps to highly sophisticated electronic equipment for performing endoscopy or injecting joints. Each activity needs clear explanations of the task to be performed. Most skills centres have experienced skills tutors from a health professions background who can help you plan the session. If they are not available, junior hospital staff and general practitioners are often able to supervise groups, as long as they are familiar with the equipment and the activities. See Chapter 5 for more information on teaching practical skills.

Students enjoy working in the non-threatening atmosphere of the skills centre where they can 'have a go', make mistakes then correct them. But, as with all teaching, a planned approach is necessary for students to make the most of the experience. Preparation will include checking that the model is functioning and all supplies are to hand. You will need to check students' knowledge and experience and plan the best use of a group's time in the centre, allocating appropriate time to each activity. Arrange a demonstration of each skill before asking students to perform it then give students constructive and immediate feedback. If the skill is complex break it down into smaller manageable parts. Ask students to practise the skill until they are comfortable and can do it fluently. This may need several sessions so you should encourage students to return to the clinical skills centre throughout their career to refresh their performance.

Communication skills suite

Whether you are teaching opportunistically, in protected time or while fulfilling service requirements you will be communicating with patients. Students will observe your communication skills and model themselves on your performance. Discussing the techniques you use to communicate with patients while actually doing so or immediately after is a powerful learning experience for students. Learning may be immediately reinforced by providing students with opportunities to practise communication skills with real patients.

Learning communication skills is a fundamental part of becoming a doctor and is as important as acquiring factual knowledge. Younger clinicians and all general practitioner registrars have learnt formally about communication and consultation skills. However many other clinicians, while adept at using consultation skills, are unfamiliar with analysing and teaching these skills.

Until recently, consultation and communication skills were not differentiated. Consultation skills are techniques we use in the medical interview (take a history, discuss management etc.), while communication skills describe how we interact with people generally. Good communication skills are essential to all aspects of medical practice and for all concerned (patients, relatives, and colleagues). The principles of teaching communication skills are covered in Chapter 5.

The use of the communications skills suites has revolutionized consultation and communication skills teaching. A typical suite contains a room where a medical interview is carried out, an observation room where a group can observe what is going on (via one-way glass or TV monitor), and video recording equipment.

Communication skills are usually taught using role play or simulated patients. The advantage of role play and simulated patients is that students can make mistakes in safety and are able to 'replay' situations until they are comfortable. To maximize learning in the communication skills suite it helps to use a standard structure:

- Set ground rules (confidentiality etc.).
- Explain the aims of the session, check prior knowledge, and explain how the session will be organized (e.g. '*First you will interview the patient for 10 minutes, then reflect on what went well and less well, and then have feedback*').
- Ask students to volunteer ("*Who would like to go first?*").
- Explain the practical task.

(*'Today you are a GP, and you are going to talk to Mr Harrison who is a 59 year old. He is a new patient, and you have 10 minutes to find out what is wrong with him and discuss how you might manage his problem.'*)

- Consider briefing students about the *content* of the consultation.

This may stop concerns about content ('I didn't know what to ask') interfering with the communication skills you want them to develop.

- Explain how the video (if available), will be used and what to do if they get stuck ('*You can ask for timeout by raising your hand*').
- Give observational tasks to the other students (e.g. '*I would like you to focus on non-verbal communication*').
- Observe the consultation along with the other students and make notes to use later.
- Feedback to the student (by the other students, simulated patient, and tutor) using segments of the video. Offer the student the chance to 'replay' difficult areas.
- Summarize and close the session.

Many medical schools have communication skills checklists that you can use as an aide memoire. Sharing your checklist with the students will help them focus their feedback. Keep feedback constructive, short, and specific. With novice students it may be helpful to follow a theme for each session; for example you might choose to look at the beginning or ending of the medical interview. With more advanced students it may be more appropriate to follow their agenda and help them with things they found difficult. Remember to use the video—actually seeing yourself in a short video clip is a powerful tool for change.

Timing is a balance between depth of feedback and maintaining the momentum of the session. If the patient interview is 10 minutes long and you plan to get feedback from the group as well, you will need to allow 20–30 minutes for each student. This may mean that you will not get through all the group in one session, so it is important to note which students have not participated to ensure that they have a go next time.

Clinical teaching without patients

You may plan a clinical session with a patient but find they are not available. If you have some notice, there are alternatives to real patients which are very useful. Their advantages and disadvantages are shown opposite.

If a patient lets you down at the last minute, arranging an alternative is much more difficult. You might consider teaching using the students and equipment you have to hand. This might include:

- Practise clinical skills (e.g. cranial nerve examination) on each other.
- Use role play to practise history taking and communication skills.
- Use available clinical resources (see opposite) to trigger a clinically orientated session.

We recommend that all clinical teachers keep a 'resource box' which contains materials to occupy students during such a session. Remove identifiers from confidential information and remember to keep adding to your box. If you keep your box up-to-date, you may be able to cover a variety of topics from cardiology to psychiatry.

A resource box for teachers

Blood test or other laboratory results.

X-rays (both normal and abnormal).

Patients case numbers (for their notes).

Copies of patient's drug chart/repeat medication form.

Pictures/quizzes from medical magazines.

Referral letters to or from hospital.

Anatomical models.

Posters and charts.

Alternative options to 'real' patients for clinical cases in your teaching

Option	Who / what are they?	Advantages	Disadvantages
Patient partners	Specially chosen and trained patients with a medical condition who 'volunteer' their time on a regular basis to teach students. Widely used with certain chronic diseases. They are usually paid expenses and a small honorarium (e.g. gift token) for their time.	Very useful for relatively stable chronic conditions, such as rheumatoid arthritis, psoriasis, or diabetes. Can give extra insights to students as experienced in their needs and often an 'expert' on their condition.	Use is mainly limited to chronic fairly stable conditions. Time-consuming to train them. Occasionally can use the session to teach students their own agenda. Some concerns about welfare of patients in repeated involvement.
Simulated patients (SP's)	These are actors or ordinary people who are trained and are employed to play the role of a patient in a scenario that you design. They therefore usually (but not always) do not have the condition they are role playing. They are used widely in OSCE exams because of the need to repeat a scenario reliably a large number of times.	Useful to ensure students are reliably getting the same experience or to fill gaps using specially designing scenarios. Very useful in exam situations to increase reliability of assessment and prevent the problem of patient fatigue. Can be interrupted and problems discussed in front of SP, who can also be trained to give feedback on student's performance.	The cost: typical fees are around £25.00 an hour, or £100 for a half-day session.Time-consuming to write good roles and train them. Students sometimes complain that they are less realistic.They are unlikely to have any relevant clinical signs.
Models	Devices include those for cardiac resuscitation, breast and pelvic examination, prostate palpation, laryngeal, eye, and ear examination, venepuncture, intravenous cannullae insertion, intra-muscular injections, catheterization, suturing, and E-T tube insertion.	Very useful for complete novice to practise skills without fear of harm. Now widely available in clinical skills centres which can be booked for teaching sessions.	Uses restricted to certain skills or practising examination techniques. Expensive to buy.
Video clips	A simple low stress way of showing students 'real' patients or scenarios they might otherwise not get direct experience of, e.g. breaking bad news. The hospital audio-visual department is often helpful in making/editing videos, or local drug rep may be able to supply one ready-made.	Useful to fill in gaps where real patient not available to students. Can demonstrate rarer signs or cases that would not otherwise be seen. Can be reassured that students all getting identical experience. Realistic as can use real patients. Can be imaginative and use excerpts from cinema films—work very well at engaging students interest.	Students can easily 'switch off' while watching unless given specific briefing (see Chapter 5). Availability of ready-made videos—can be expensive to buy. Issues of consent for using videos of real patients in teaching.
Paper case vignettes	A low tech option useful to have prepared as a back-up in case of disaster. Can be done direct from case notes, or pre-prepared by you to highlight key features. Important to be based on 'real' case rather than idealized 'classical' case.	Cheap, fairly easy to prepare. Can be realistic if based on real patients. Easy to integrate into seminar or large group lecture setting.	Can lack realism, especially if it is a'classical case'. Can be difficult to write a good case. Can not use to practise skills, e.g. examination techniques.

Conclusion

Learning in the clinical setting is very important and interesting for students but can be difficult for teachers who have to balance teaching, clinical care, and administrative commitments. Sometimes it is possible teach in protected time but much teaching has to go on amid clinical work. Keep a resource box to use if your patient fails to turn up. To make the most of clinical learning agree clear objectives at the beginning of the session, focus learning on agreed tasks, encourage all the students to participate, and observe student performance with feedback. At the end of each session however short or opportunistic, encourage students to summarize and reflect on their experience before planning how to reinforce learning by further practice.

References

Cox, K. (1993) Planning bedside teaching. *Med J Aust* **158**, 280–2.

DaRosa, D. A., Dunnington, G. L., Stearns, J., Ferenchick, G., Bowen, J. L., and Simpson, D. E. (1997) Ambulatory teaching "lite": less clinic time, more educationally fulfilling. *Acad Med* **72**, 358–61.

Ferenchick, G., Simpson, D., Blackman, J., DaRosa, D., and Dunnington, G. (1997) Strategies for efficient and effective teaching in the ambulatory care setting. *Acad Med* **72**, 277–80.

Flexner, A. (1910) *Medical education in the United States and Canada: a report to the Carnegie Foundation for the advancement of teaching.* Bulletin No 4. Boston MA: Updyke.

Harth, S. C., Bavanandan, S., Thomas, K. E., Lai, M. Y., and Thong, Y. H. (1992) The quality of student–tutor interactions in the clinical learning environment. *Med Educ* **26**, 321–6.

Heidenreich, C., Lye, P., Simpson, D., and Lourich, M. (2000) The search for effective and efficient ambulatory teaching methods through the literature. *Pediatrics* **105**, 231–7.

Irby, D. M. (1995) Teaching and learning in ambulatory care settings: a thematic review of the literature. *Acad Med* **70**, 898–931.

Laidley, T. L., Braddock, C. H., and Fihn, S. D. (2000) Did I answer your question? Attending physicians' recognition of residents' perceived learning needs in ambulatory settings. *J Gen Intern Med* **15**, 46–50.

Malley, P. G., Kroenke, K., Ritter, J., Dy, N., and Pangaro, L. (1999) What learners and teachers value most in ambulatory educational encounters: a prospective, qualitative study. *Acad Med* **74**, 186–91.

Mann, K. V., Holmes, D. B., Hayes, V. M., Burge, F. I., and Viscount, P. W. (2001) Community family medicine teachers' perceptions of their teaching role. *Med Educ* **35**, 278–85.

Neher, J. O., Gordan, K. A., Meyer, B., and Stevens, N. (1992) A 5 step microskills model of clinical teaching. *J Am Board Fam Pract* **5**, 419–24.

Newble, D., and Cannon, R. (1994) *A handbook for medical teachers*, 3rd edn. London: Kluwer Academic Publishers.

Skeff, K. M., Bowen, J. L., and Irby, D. M. (1997) Protecting time for teaching in the ambulatory care setting. *Acad Med* **72**, 694–7.

Usatine, R. P., Tremoulet, P. T., and Irby, D. (2000) Time-efficient preceptors in ambulatory care settings. *Acad Med* **75**, 639–42.

CHAPTER 9

Designing a course

'The kids we bring into medical school are wonderful with the highest possible qualities. We then submerge them in facts and beat the imagination out of them.'

K. Calman, 1997

No matter how wonderful your individual teaching session is, it will be affected by the other sessions on the course. Designing a course and making sure it works well takes a lot of time and effort, but the underlying principles are straightforward, and useful for all teachers. In this chapter we will look at how to design a course and some of the underlying principle and ideas.

What is a course?

A course is generally understood to mean a series of learning experiences centred round a topic. Within teaching you are likely to find that the words course, programme, syllabus, and curriculum are used interchangeably.

Definitions

Course—colloquial term used for anything from a one week ENT attachment to the entire medical school curriculum.

Programme—often used in US publications, tends to refer to a limited period of study in one topic area.

Syllabus—the (often written) statement of the content of the course. This may be framed in terms of objectives or outcomes.

Curriculum—this embraces not only the content but also the teaching strategies and delivery of the teaching programme.

Not all of a course is planned—some things are not learned despite being taught while others, like attitudes, may be learned informally. The latter situation is often referred to as '**the hidden curriculum**'. This hidden learning is entirely off syllabus and may even be undesirable—the negative attitudes that many students acquire during medical school are a good example. Some of the planned course may not be taught, and some teachers may not teach all of it. This mismatch between planning, learning, and teaching is shown in figure 29.

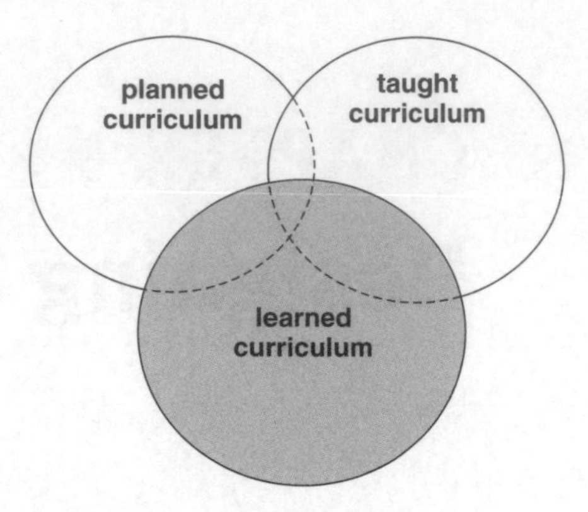

Figure 9.1 Mismatch between planning, learning, and teaching

In an ideal world all the circles would perfectly overlap. In practice, the more overlap we manage, the better we are doing.

Most courses are not just about content and the way that it is delivered: they also have an assessment to make sure that the students have learned the content. Ideally a course should be balanced, in that the objectives should be evenly represented in the course content and assessment. In real life imbalances often occur between objectives, course content, and assessment.

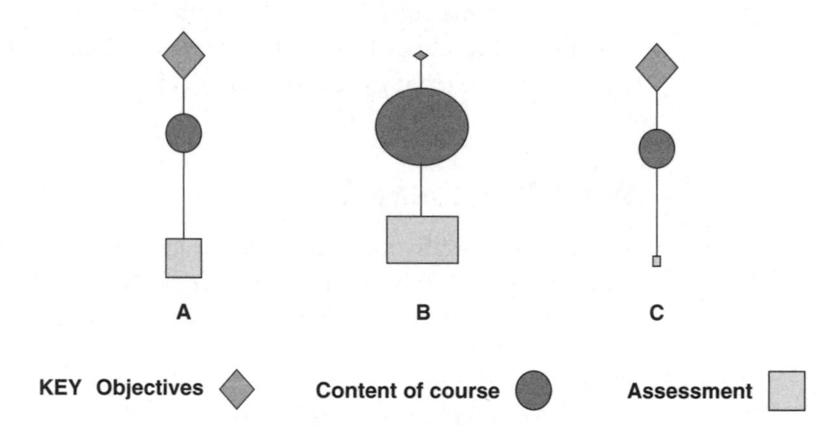

Figure 9.2 Balancing objectives, course content, and assessment

The ideal course should look like A in the diagram above, where the objectives of the course match the taught course content and the assessment exactly. B represents the situation in many UK medical schools until recently, where there were few objectives, a large taught course, and an assessment which did not always reflect either the course or the objectives. Finally, it is also common to find well designed courses which are little assessed—C. This can be demotivating for students.

In the medical setting it is fairly rare to have the responsibility of developing a wholly new course. This does happen from time to time, but it is more common to inherit the mangement of an already developed course. It is perfectly possible to continue with the same content and teaching methods for years, but even if the course was perfectly designed to begin with it will rapidly become rather threadbare. In real life courses are '**dynamic**'—that is to say they do not stay the same. You will have new teachers, changes in student numbers, positive or negative feedback from students, and an evolving content as medicine advances. You will probably want to try new things and leave a personal stamp on the course.

Sometimes managing a course feels like running to stand still. The amount of running is directly related to the amount of innovation you decide to impose, and it is wise to check whether your administrator and fellow teachers are fit for a marathon before you start.

Devising a new course

Getting started

If you are planning to start afresh, or extensively overhaul an existing programme, the first question that you should ask yourself is what the course is intended to cover. This may not be the same as its actual content, and you may have to refer back to the original curriculum documents. Any changes to the course content will need to go through the appropriate curriculum committee.

Getting a course off the ground is a lot of work. It will take you a minimum of six months, and it will be helpful if you can get a group of teachers and administrative staff in your field together, and form a course committee. If you plan some radical developments it is advisable to seek early advice from your medical education unit and the curriculum committee. The structure of your course committee will depend on your personality—some course leaders prefer an informal structure, while others will head for a more formal arrangement. Whatever the structure of your committee, it is important to ensure that you record your meetings and keep all pertinent information together. Not only will this make running the course easier, but it will be enormously helpful for future course evaluation.

Once you have convened your group, you can start to create your course. The key steps for you to follow are:

(a) To define the content.

(b) To organize the content.

(c) To select the teaching methods.

(d) To organize assessment.

(e) To evaluate the course.

(f) To feedback the evaluation into the next course.

This circularity is rather like the audit cycle, and can be shown below. Continually re-evaluating and re-constructing a course is the best way to keep it up-to-date and fresh.

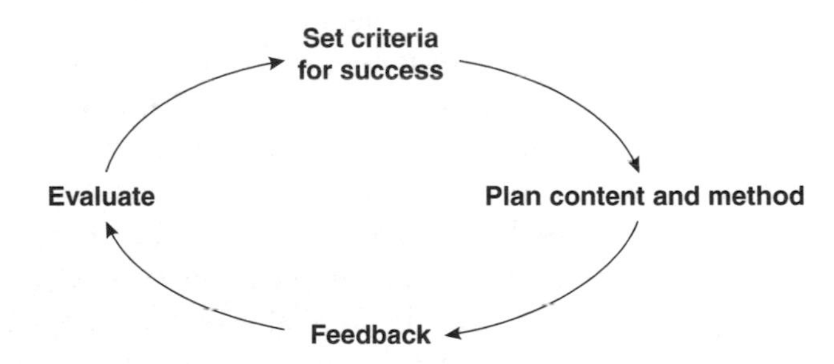

Figure 9.3 The course development cycle

Defining the content

If the course content is not defined you will need to set it. There are two basic ways of doing this. First, you could approach it from the point of view of medical teachers or specialists in the appropriate clinical field. The problem with this approach is that you are likely to end up with a lot of content. The alternative approach is to consider what a junior doctor needs to be able to do on the wards. This will automatically reduce the content, but may go too far in the other direction, and leave your medical students with gaps in their knowledge.

Once the key '**outcomes**' (the knowledge or tasks required) have been identified (Harden *et al.*, 1999; Dunn *et al.*, 1985), then the content can be defined backwards from these. You may choose to state your content as objectives or as competencies (see Chapter 2). Some of the content you have defined may already be covered on different courses—checking with other course leaders is vital.

In any course, some of the content is absolutely essential for all doctors and is considered to be '**core**'. Other information may be less essential, and you might want to offer it to students in the form of '**options**' (Harden and Davis, 1995). Many courses feel crowded as the 'core' content continues to expand. Taking a critical look at it may help you free up some time.

Organizing the content

Once the content is clear you will need to decide how to organize it. You may decide to cover key basics first and then move on to their clinical applications, or to use clinical experiences from the start. What you decide to do will depend on what the students already know, where in the curriculum you are, how much time you have at your disposal, and what assessments you plan to use. It is helpful to write down the content list, and see whether you can link certain topics together, and whether information in one topic is essential for the understanding of another.

You may choose to go through each subject to the depth required using a '**linear**' approach (appropriate for a shorter course) or to repeatedly revisit subjects, looking at them in greater depth each time. This latter approach is often called the '**spiral curriculum**' (Bruner, 1966).

Whichever you choose it is important to make sure that students have the essential pre-learning in place to make sense of the new information, and are presented with the information in a logical manner.

Historical sources show that medical students learned in a haphazard fashion, supplementing apprenticeships with occasional lectures (Porter, 1997). The development of systematic teaching in the basic sciences proposed by Flexner was a revolutionary idea (Tyler, 1950), which eventually spread to all medical schools. These early medical curricula were taught in a linear fashion—that is to say they started with the basic sciences, and then moved on to clinical study. The advantage of this system was felt to be that students would thoroughly understand the basic sciences and then be able to use them in clinical work. However, subsequent experience showed that this system tended to lead to redundancy, curricular overload, and knowledge that did not integrate easily with clinical work (General Medical Council, 1993). New models of teaching medicine were developed which used an integrated approach in which the relevant basic sciences were integrated with clinical information and presented to the students. Integration can be described as either **vertical** (in which the basic sciences are integrated with clinical experience) or **horizontal** (in which different basic sciences are mixed together) (Harden *et al.*, 1984). The systems approach is horizontal integration, while early clinical experience is vertical integration. Other changes have reduced the curriculum overload by defining the 'core' content of the medical curriculum and allowing students to select 'electives' in which they wished further information.

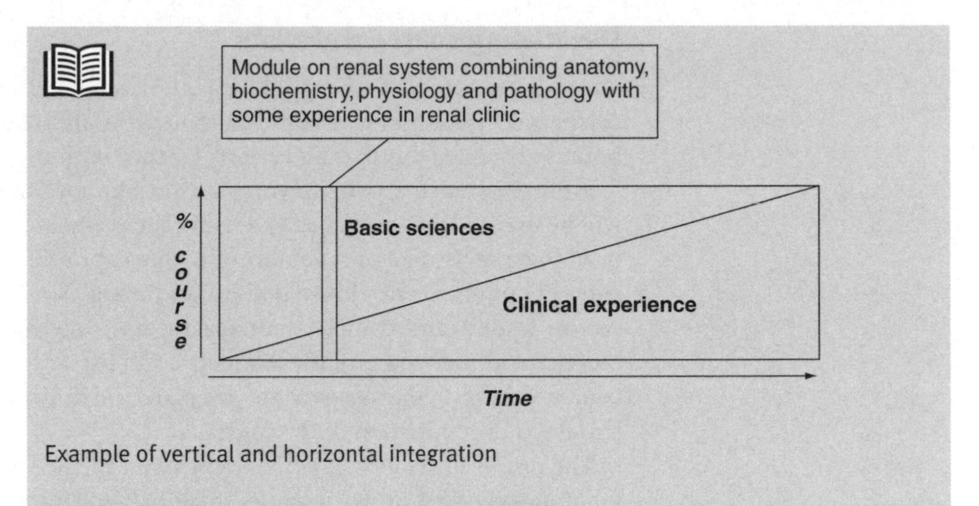

Example of vertical and horizontal integration

An example of vertical and horizontal integration. During the course the students increase the amount of time they spend on clinical experience, and a systems style approach is used where students learn all the relevant sciences related to one organ system at a time.

Choosing the teaching methods

By now you should have a structured idea of the information you want to get across and the order in which this should be done. The next question to consider is how to get this information across. Some decisions are guided by the nature of the information you are trying to get across—for example, practical skills have to be taught in the skills laboratory or at the bedside. Other decisions depend on the students—for example, their likely mix of learning styles means it is wise to offer a mixture of teaching techniques. Think laterally, and don't be afraid to try out new techniques. It may be helpful to talk to other course leaders about what teaching methods they have used and build on particularly successful ideas. Ultimately many decisions will be affected by administration: the numbers of students you have to teach, the available teaching staff, and the practical resources (rooms, etc.).

This does not mean that you should rule out some teaching techniques, but you may need to be creative in your application of them. It may be impossible to move to a fully PBL course (you haven't got the staff or the space) but perhaps you could introduce a couple of cases into your teaching this year. If you get wonderful evaluations, you may be able to gradually increase the PBL content over time.

Timetabling

This is a complex task. You will need an efficient administrator, precise information from the medical school on the number of students and the dates of the attachment, as well as an idea of the potential availability of your teachers and resources. It may be wise to construct a preliminary grid on which you map out the potential resources (e.g. rooms, ward rounds, outpatient clinics) and teachers available each am and pm, along with the order of the course content. You will rapidly see whether the small group work that you planned for the second half of Week 2 will need to take place in Week 3. Try several possible drafts and talk them through with your course group. Remember that the first few courses are likely to be rather rocky, and you will need to be flexible if something is not working out.

Once the order of the course has been decided it is very important to book rooms, inform clinicians of their likely involvement, and start to get the course material prepared.

Developing course materials

You will need to think about course materials for both your students and for your teachers. The course materials need to be clear and relevant. It helps to have them bound or stapled together and clearly labelled with the name of the course.

From the students' point of view, the most important part of the course materials will be the student timetable, which tells them where they are going to be. This will need to be revised before the start of each rotation. If students need to travel, consider giving them travel instructions and maps. Students will need details of the course leaders and contact numbers in case they have difficulties. We strongly recommend that you give the students a full list of the aims and objectives of the course, details on the assessments you plan, and information on how they can contribute to the evaluation of the course.

The rest of the course materials depend on the needs of the course. If you plan a lot of independent study, the course materials will have to be very precise, otherwise they may consist of a series of handouts from lectures, pre-reading for seminars, recommended reading lists, and practical problems to work through.

Your teachers will need a copy of the student course guide. In addition they also need detailed objectives for each session, and (if appropriate) teaching plans. If you want your teachers to prepare the students for an end-of-course assessment, they will need information about the assessments and sample questions.

Presentation of the course materials depends on the resources of the department. Loose leaf files, photocopied pages, and even CD-ROMs can be used. Make sure that you have sufficient administration support to produce your materials and that there will be enough for all the students.

Developing your teachers

Telling the students what they are going to do will be of little use if your teachers are unprepared. The amount of staff development you will need to do depends on the degree of innovation you have planned and the quality of evaluations you have had about the teaching in the past. The first step is to inform everyone of what you plan. There are many ways to do this, but we recommend telling everyone in person—either one at a time, or at a meeting. This allows your teachers to discuss the plans and see how they will fit into them. Once the plans are clear, you can ask people what skills and resources they would need to deliver them. Areas of need can be identified and you can ask your teachers what they think would help them to learn the skills required. You will be able to get help from your medical education unit to train your teachers.

Spearheading any major curriculum change requires considerable personal drive and leadership. Don't be surprised if your teachers seem to be obstructive. Gentle, good humoured persistence and well-marshalled arguments will eventually erode the most persistent of your detractors.

All curriculum development requires change. The process of change can be either evolutionary or revolutionary. The adoption of new teaching strategies over the past few decades has varied hugely from institution to institution, with some being 'innovators' while others adopt late if at all. The key to adopting an innovation is finding a 'change agent' who enthusiastically promotes it. The change agent will face a series of institutional barriers (Mennin and Kaufman, 1989), including concerns about losing control, the cost of the innovation, wasting time on something not associated with promotion, and a feeling that the *status quo* is perfectly adequate.

To overcome resistance, it is worth considering the following (Grant and Gale, 1989):

1 Demonstrating the need for change.
2 Involving stake-holders in the change process.
3 Providing information and encouragement.
4 Making future plans clear.
5 Enlisting key people to ensure support for the change.
6 Postponing or accelerating events if necessary.
7 Providing staff development to cope with the change.

Once the change is in place, sustaining it requires the constructive use of evaluation and ongoing enthusiasm.

Planning the assessment

The way in which you assess the course will influence the way in which your students learn. More detail on assessment is found in Chapter 10. You will be assessing your students both formatively and summatively. You may have little control over the summative assessment—for example the students may have an end-of-year exam to which you will be asked to contribute some MCQs, but you are likely to have a free hand with the formative assessment and the possibility of trying new approaches. Working with your course team will spread the work, and give you new ideas.

The first stage of devising an assessment is to decide what areas of the course are to be assessed, and ensure that you cover the course fairly. You will then want to choose the assessment techniques, decide on standards, write the questions, and produce some model answers. Finally, you will need to recruit and train markers, and evaluate the assessment.

There are plenty of techniques that you can use in formative assessment. You may want to consider whether your assessment is to be continuous or a 'snapshot' (end-of-course examination), and whether you want to assess individuals or the group. Think about using feedback sessions, logbooks, case presentations, project work, and portfolios. Your students will enjoy new approaches and will be encouraged to work throughout the course.

Planning the evaluation

If courses were delivered exactly as planned, the role of the evaluator would be much easier. You will want to see whether the course delivered the original aims and how far it departed from what was planned. To find out what actually went on you will have to ask those who experienced and delivered the course—students, teachers, and administrators. The best evaluations are those that are planned from the inception of the course. Work with your course team, think about the key questions you want answered, and devise your evaluation around them. More information on constructing evaluations is found in Chapter 11.

Evaluations always turn up surprises, and it is important to have enough information to understand what actually went on. It is tempting to rely on questionnaires completed by students and staff, but remember that a score of 2 (poor) will not tell you what the problems were. The first few times you run a course, and after any major changes, try discuss the course with staff and students towards the end of the attachment. Ask them what the good points were, what didn't work too well, and how things could be improved. Ten minutes chat will give you a far more balanced view of the strengths and weaknesses of the course than two hours poring over a stack of evaluation forms. Once the course has matured you may want to move to using evaluation forms. A mixture of rating scales and open-ended questions will give you the best information. Evaluation forms which are not completed are no help at all. Give one of your administration staff the responsibility of getting the forms out and back in again. It may be possible to link receipt of the forms with signing off at the end of the course.

Delivering your first course

After all your work, you will be ready to deliver the first course. This is always an anxious time, and it may help to have a timeline in mind to help you get a course off the ground. A typical development timeline for a medium-sized course is shown below.

Time	Tasks
> Six months pre-course	Convene course team of teacher and administrators to present need for change and essential information (student numbers, how the course will fit in with the curriculum).
	Discuss course content—seek opinions of other teachers and curriculum committee.
Six months pre-course	Course meeting to agree course content, organization of content, and teaching methods. Apportion roles within course team: responsibility for content, course materials, assessment, and evaluation.
	Devise assessment and evaluation.
	Start to write course materials.
	Check plans with curriculum committee and medical education unit.
	Use resources grid to plan delivery of course.
Three months pre-course	Book rooms.
	General meeting to inform all staff and perform needs assessment for teachers and administrators.
Two months pre-course	Plan staff development.
One month pre-course	Circulate timetable to all teaching staff, and check that they are available.
One week pre-course	Ensure enough course materials are available, and double-check that all staff know what they are doing.
During course	Remember to administer assessment and evaluations.
End of course	Communicate assessment results to students, teachers, and medical school.
One–two months post-course	Feedback evaluation results (and write course report if required) to teachers, course team, and to curriculum committee, with details of planned changes for next course.

Final steps

A week before you go live, double-check student numbers and resource availability. Make sure that your teachers all know what they are teaching, where and when; that the course materials are adequate; and that assessment and evaluation tools are ready and securely stored. Check that the course leaders (you are likely to be one) have a full list of the students, and that any special information about any of the students has been appropriately disseminated.

The first session

If you have not done so already, you will need to consider how you open the course. The first session is very important, and will set the standard for the rest of the course. One of the most common complaints about courses is that communication was inadequate at the start. Try and use the most welcoming venue that you can find to start off, and, if your budget will stretch, offer the students tea and coffee. Welcome the students, introduce everyone, and clearly lay out what they can expect from the course and what you expect of them. If you want the students to use different learning resources, either walking them around your department or offering a map will help. Finally, make sure that they know who to contact if there are problems, and how you will contact them in emergency. It may be helpful to ask one of the students to act as the chief contact. Keep the first session relatively short, and if possible keep the learning load down on the first day. Your students will be tired from all the new information, and you will be tired from the accumulated stress of the past few weeks.

What students need to know about a course (adapted from Dent and Harden, 2001)

- What they should be learning—the detailed course objectives/outcomes.
- The depth to which they will need to study—the standard required.
- What range of learning experiences and opportunities are available.
- How and when they can access these—the timetable.
- How they will be assessed, and what will happen if they don't pass.
- Who to turn to if they need help.
- How the course will be evaluated.

Monitoring progress

Try and meet with the students in the middle of the course to check that everything is going well, and arrange to meet them again at the end. Make sure that the assessment and evaluations are completed, and the results communicated to the students.

Students on the first run-through of a course often complain that they feel like guinea pigs. We tend to underestimate the importance of the medical school 'grapevine' in telling students what to expect from a course, and deprived of the accumulated experience of their peers, students can feel very lost. They will have serious concerns about whether new teaching techniques will damage their learning, and whether they will be disadvantaged compared with their peers who took the previous course. This can lead to some difficult experiences for teachers and students alike. Try and address their issues openly at the start of the course. Acknowledge that there will be difficulties, and if possible try and operate an 'open-door' policy to deal with grievances before they become serious.

Managing subsequent courses

After all your work, you will want to sit back and let subsequent courses run themselves. Unfortunately things tend not to work out like that. The major hurdle will be over but anticipate a year of teething difficulties before the course has really settled down. The difficulty with this is that major curriculum upheavals tend to sap the strength of even the most committed innovator, and you may wonder if you have the enthusiasm to keep going in the face of problems. Your task will be made much easier if you develop good administrative systems, and have an efficient teaching administrator. Try and delegate as much of the day-to-day running of the course as you can, and see your eventual role as dealing with the academic and teaching problems that arise. A good course will be continually evolving, and you will want to keep innovating. Remember the other teachers in the team. They may also be tired out by the change. Think about supporting them with ongoing staff development and meetings to discuss progress.

Revising existing courses

Medicine is continually changing, and as a result all courses need to be regularly revised. Medical schools should have quality assurance processes in place to make sure that this happens. In practice an approach of 'If it ain't broke, don't fix it' is common. This leads to complaints from medical students, who are very vocal about the quality of their medical education, and good at detecting when courses are getting rusty.

Intervening only when courses start to fail leads to a backwards looking attitude to course development. It does not disseminate good practice, but leads to a focus on problems and identification of failing teachers. The resultant blame culture is divisive and unhelpful. It is much more positive to continually update courses.

If you are asked to revise a course it is helpful to follow the standard procedure for developing a new course while bearing in mind at each step:

(a) Where the course is with regard to objectives/content/assessment.

(b) Where the faculty want the course to be.

(c) How to get there.

Revising a course is a delicate time for current staff, who may have invested much time and work in the current course. Major revisions affect teaching and administration staff, and managing the process of change may be difficult and tiring. By focusing on the positive, looking forward, and following the structured approach outlined above you will be able to make the necessary changes and improvements without further sapping morale.

Curricula and courses can be analysed in several dimensions, relating to the way in which information is organized and delivered. One of the most quoted is the SPICES model (Harden *et al.*, 1984). This is shown below:

Student centred	↔	Teacher centred
Problem based	↔	Information gathering
Integrated	↔	Discipline based
Community based	↔	Hospital based
Elective	↔	Uniform
Systematic	↔	Apprenticeship based

Twenty years ago nearly all medical schools were very much to the right of each of the spectra, with traditional, teacher centred, discipline-based curricula. Teaching was centred round the hospital, and a lot of the learning used the apprenticeship model. Medicine has changed and now medical schools mostly occupy the centre left of the spectrum. Curricula are more integrated, a 'core' curricula for medicine has been identified and students are encouraged to study elective subjects in more depth. Teaching has become more student centred, particularly in schools that have a problem-based curriculum. Medical school are all different and there is no one position on the spectra which is 'best'. It is likely that being at either extreme end of the spectra is uncomfortable for the majority of students.

Conclusion

Planning a new course is hugely rewarding, but is hard work. You can spread your load by working with a group of committed teachers. With your group, set a timeline and build your course, assessment, and evaluation at the same time. This will ensure that the content and assessment match up and that you have feedback mechanisms in place to keep your course dynamic. Remember that the first few courses will be far from perfect and expect to adjust the course until it runs smoothly.

References

Bruner, J. (1966) *Towards a theory of instruction.* Cambridge Mass.: Harvard University Press.

Dent, J. A., and Harden, R. (2001) *A practical guide for medical teachers.* Edinburgh: Churchill Livingstone.

Dunn, W. R., Hamilton, D. D., and Harden, R. M. (1985) Techniques for identifying competencies needed of doctors. *Med Teach* **1**, 15–25.

General Medical Council. (1993) *Tomorrow's doctors. Recommendations on undergraduate medical education.* General Medical Council, London.

Grant, J., and Gale, R. (1989) Changing medical education. *Med Educ* **23**, 252–7.

Harden, R. M., and Davis, M. (1995) The core curriculum with options or special study modules. *Med Educ* **29**, 125–48.

Harden, R., Crosby, J., and Davies, M. H. (1999) *AMEE medical education guide No 14: Outcome-based education.* Dundee: AMEE.

Harden, R. M., Sowden, S., and Dunn, W. R. (1984) Some educational strategies in curriculum development: the SPICES model. *Med Educ* **18**, 284–97.

Mennin, S., and Kaufman, A. (1989) The change process and medical education. *Med Teach* **11**, 9–16.

Porter, R. (1997) *The greatest benefit to mankind: a medical history of humanity from antiquity to the present.* London: Harper Collins.

Tyler, R. W. (1950) *Basic principles of curriculum and instruction.* Chicago: University of Chicago Press.

Further reading

Dent, J. A., and Harden, R. (2001) *A practical guide for medical teachers.* Edinburgh: Churchill Livingstone.

CHAPTER 10

Assessing students

Assessment is about getting to know our students and the quality of their learning.
Rowntree, 1977

What is assessment?

All of us get involved in assessments because we want to know how much our students have learned. However many of us perceive student assessment to be difficult and confusing. This seems to be because assessment has a complicated jargon, and several new and unfamiliar techniques. We also appreciate that assessment is a high stakes business, and don't want to get involved in making mistakes that could have catastrophic results for our students.

It is true that some assessments can be very important for students and powerfully influence the way they learn. We need to design assessments carefully. Results need to be fair and accurate, but they should also be defensible, as students are increasingly likely to challenge the results. An interest in improving accuracy has led to the development of a precise language to describe assessment, and to new assessment techniques. However the underlying principles of assessment are not complicated. The first half of the chapter looks at some of the theory behind assessment, while the second half looks in detail at the different techniques of assessment you and your students might face.

Assessment versus evaluation

In the UK, the accepted definitions are:

Assessment: measuring how much the learner has learned.

Evaluation: measuring the quality of teaching. This might be your teaching, your course, or the whole institution.

Many teachers use these terms imprecisely, and literature from other countries may use 'student evaluation' where we would use 'assessment'.

Types of assessment

There are two types of assessment, depending on how you plan to use the information gathered.

Summative assessment

This will be familiar to you from your days as a student. It is used to make formal decisions about whether a learner has achieved a set standard. It usually takes place at the end of a course, is often expressed as a mark or grade, and is not something you want to fail. Examples would include end-of-firm assessments, end-of-year examinations, medical finals, and professional qualifications (e.g. MRCP or MRCGP). Summative assessment uses a variety of assessment techniques, which you may become directly involved with, or need to be familiar with to help your students prepare for them.

Formative assessment

This is used by all teachers all the time, although they may not use the term. It means looking at a learner's progress in an informal way, with the aim of helping the learner towards a particular goal. An example would be setting a quick test at the end of a session to check how much your learners have taken in. You would then offer them feedback on their performance, and advice on how to reach the expected standard.

There is obviously quite a bit of overlap between the two types. For example, some medical schools use end-of-firm assessments formatively, while others use them summatively. Once the type of assessment has been chosen, you can select from an array of assessment techniques which measure the learners performance.

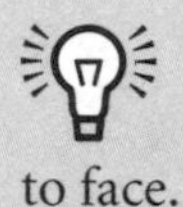

About to be a marker for the first time? Read *Who does the assessment—teachers* followed by the section on the type of assessment you are due to face.

Why do we assess students?

Assessment is vital for good teaching and learning. At a formative level, you might use assessment information to see what level your students have reached, and to find out whether they have any particular learning problems. Sharing this information with the students helps them to understand what they need to do to improve, which is why simply giving a bald 3/10 result for a piece of work is unhelpful. Using a more detailed approach to marking helps you to alter your teaching to meet their needs and to help them pass their next examination. The information would also be useful to provide you with some feedback on your own teaching—next time you might think about checking whether the students understood the theory beforehand, slow the pace a little, or alter your teaching strategies.

Summative assessment is vital in ensuring that students who graduate from medical school are competent doctors. Because it is very important to medical students and medical schools, it gets a lot of attention. However it has the side-effect of driving both the content and strategy of student learning. Thus once students know the content they are likely to be examined on, they will target their learning towards that. This can be useful—important, but previously neglected subjects can suddenly fill lecture theatres once their presence in a summative assessment is announced. The assessment technique will drive the learning strategy used by students. Thus if your clinical placements are assessed by a written examination, do not be surprised if students spend the last two weeks of a firm in the library rather than in clinic.

Summative assessment is a time-consuming, expensive, and difficult process to do well. It is a high stakes occupation for all the participants. The learners have their professional future at stake, the teachers have their reputation as effective teachers, and the institution is vulnerable to legal challenge if the process is felt to be inaccurate or unfair.

The use of summative assessment has been challenged within higher education, with many debates about its ill effects (Curzon, 1994). The arguments revolve around two key areas. First, assessment places constraints on the written syllabus, on the freedom that teachers have to interpret the syllabus, and may drive the learning of the students in deleterious ways. Within medicine we would argue that the profession and society require doctors that are competent in certain areas, and that this both constrains the syllabus and requires summative assessment to ensure that standards are met. In order to drive learning in positive ways we need to select assessment techniques that are appropriate. Secondly, assessment (or rather failure in assessments) can lead to anxiety and low esteem in learners. While this is true, concealing such information from learners, or implying that it is not important, may be doing them a disservice in later life. Dealing with anxiety induced by examinations requires preparing learners, and for this the use of formative assessment is vital.

Due to their importance, summative assessment often overshadows formative assessments, and may even come to dominate teaching. However formative assessment is very beneficial to the learner. To be successful both students and teacher need to share a common view of what is to be achieved, the assessment needs to be carefully planned, and good quality feedback is essential (Dent and Harden, 2001).

'Realistic awareness of our relative intellectual status among our peers is a fact of life to which all of us must eventually adjust and the sooner the better for everyone concerned. There is no profit in sugar-coating the truth or self-delusion' (Ausubel et al., 1978).

Who does the assessment?

Until recently it was assumed that all assessment should be done by teachers. However the use of self-assessment and peer assessment is becoming more popular.

The teachers

The benefits of assessment by teachers are that we know the students, we know the syllabus, and understand the standards that students have to meet. However in the real world we often have many students at any one time, and may lack the time to assess each student completely. It is appropriate in a 'high stakes' assessment that a teacher takes part, if only because they are more likely to be seen as impartial by the students. At the formative level your assessment is key to helping your students overcome difficulties with their learning, particularly if you will need to make some changes in the course. The key to making the most of formative assessment is high quality feedback to the students, as outlined in Chapter 4.

For an assessment to be fair, the examiners must be seen to mark every student on their merits, and not be biased. This '**objectivity**' is easier if examiners use a checklist or marksheet on which they record whether a behaviour has been observed or not. Training or the use of two markers may further reduce bias.

A pre-exam checklist for examiners

- **Organization.** Where and at what time am I assessing the students?
- **Standards.** What level should the students be at?
- **Content.** What areas of the syllabus (aims and objectives) and what domains (knowledge, skills, and attitudes) am I expected to cover?
- **Examination.** What type of assessment instruments will be used and do I know how to use them?

Preparing for summative assessments

Examiners need to be prepared. If asked to formally assess students make sure you are clear about the type of exam involved. If you have not marked a similar exam before, ask if it is possible for you to sit in on one. It is helpful to talk to your colleagues, ask to see old questions or sample marking papers, and make sure that you know the standard students are expected to reach. Check that you are clear about the organization—you may need to be there early to set up or brief the students before the start. If you are expected to do the timekeeping, check that you have a working timer or watch.

Increasing the objectivity of examiners has been tackled by developing objective marking schedules, and by training. The two forms of objective marking schedules are checklists and rating scales. Checklists note whether a behaviour has been observed or not while rating scales require a value judgement about the degree to which something has been achieved. They are undoubtedly helpful for inexperienced examiners, and of particular use in self-assessment and peer assessment. There are six common errors made by examiners when using rating scales (Guilford, 1974).

1 **Leniency**. Some examiners ('doves') mark higher than others, and this may occur in isolation if the examiner likes the candidate.
2 **Central tendency**. Most examiners only use the middle points of the scale.
3 **Halo effect**. The examiner's overall opinion of the student influences his marking of a specific trait.
4 **Logical error**. Similar scores are often given to two things which seem to be related.
5 **Proximity errors**. Similar scores to related traits occur particularly if they are close together on the form.
6 **Contrast errors**. Expert examiners tend to mark harder in their own field than elsewhere.

Rating scales can be designed that address some of these problems by providing clear instructions, defining exactly what is expected of a student who is awarded an A, B, or C, and adjusting the scale to compensate for the central tendency. Using more than one examiner increases objectivity.

While the evidence that training examiners increases objectivity is equivocal, it is good practice for institutions to provide it (Fry *et al.*, 1999).

The students (self-assessment)

For students to become lifelong learners they need to be able to accurately assess their own performance. This is a skill, and like all skills improves with practise. Letting students assess their own performance, and then feeding back to them on your assessment of their performance will improve their accuracy. Examples of self-assessment include multiple choice questions at the end of chapters in books (with answers at the back) and asking students to rate their competence in clinical skills.

Making self-assessment work

Getting self-assessment to work is harder than it may appear, and for it to be a success, you need to consider the points below (Dent and Harden, 2001).

Making self-assessment work

1 **Aim** to enhance learning.

2 **Clarify** the aims of the exercise and what will be required with the students.

3 **Make** it voluntary.

4 **Keep** other forms of assessment in place (if students think that you will use the information summatively they may distort the results).

5 **Involve** the students in setting the criteria, make sure that they are clearly defined, measureable, and written down in a usable format.

6 **Ensure** good rapport with the students beforehand.

7 **Feedback** in detail to students on their performance.

Other students (peer assessment)

Peer assessment means that students assess each other. They should be able to mark each other and then to justify the marks that they award. Many of the points about self-assessment also apply to peer assessment, with the additional complexity that you need to be able to manage the group dynamics.

What makes a good assessment?

A good assessment needs to accurately determine the depth and breadth of learning that a student has achieved, and be seen to be just by faculty and students.

Your assessment should reflect the learning that has taken place. This is easier if you have designed the course around clear objectives, and tailored the assessment to test these objectives. Students have successfully challenged assessments in the courts in the USA on the basis that the assessment did not reflect the taught course (McManus, 1998, quoted in Fry *et al.*, 1999).

It is also important that your assessment is accurate. An accurate assessment needs to be **reliable** and **valid**, but it won't be used unless it is **feasible**, i.e. not too time-consuming, expensive, or labour-intensive. The concepts of reliability and validity are key to assessment and are looked at in more detail below.

Reliability

This means that if a student sat the same test on two different occasions, they would get a similar mark. The higher the reliability of an assessment, the more confidence you can have in the result. The most reliable tests (e.g. multiple choice questions or MCQs) contain many items which test a wide field of content, and do not involve an examiner. This is because examiners often lack '**objectivity**'. They can be influenced by students' anxiety, personal bias, or they may only question students on their pet topic. Examiners may be referred to as 'hawks' who are hard to please, or 'doves', who pass everyone. As a result some traditional forms of assessment (e.g. essays or orals) are less reliable. Increasing examiner objectivity is helped the use of marking schedules and training (Dent and Harden, 2001).

Factors affecting reliability

Length. More items per test increase reliability.

Objectivity. The more objective the examiner can be the higher the reliability. This is particularly important in marking essay questions and orals. Use of a marking schedule and examiner training may improve reliability.

Environment. Must be appropriate for the type of test.

Processing errors. Care should be taken in calculating scores.

Not only do test techniques vary in their reliability, but so do students. Another use of the term reliability refers to the consistency of student performance across different cases—'**intercase reliability**'. All of us have some areas of practice where we are less competent than others, and if a short examination assessed us on only areas in which we had difficulty, it might conclude that we were incompetent. To make sure that you have really assessed a student's competence you need many questions, making assessments longer. Longer examinations have different intercase reliability, as shown below (Wass *et al.*, 2001).

From this it can be seen that MCQs have the highest intercase reliability, as might be expected from an objective test with many questions.

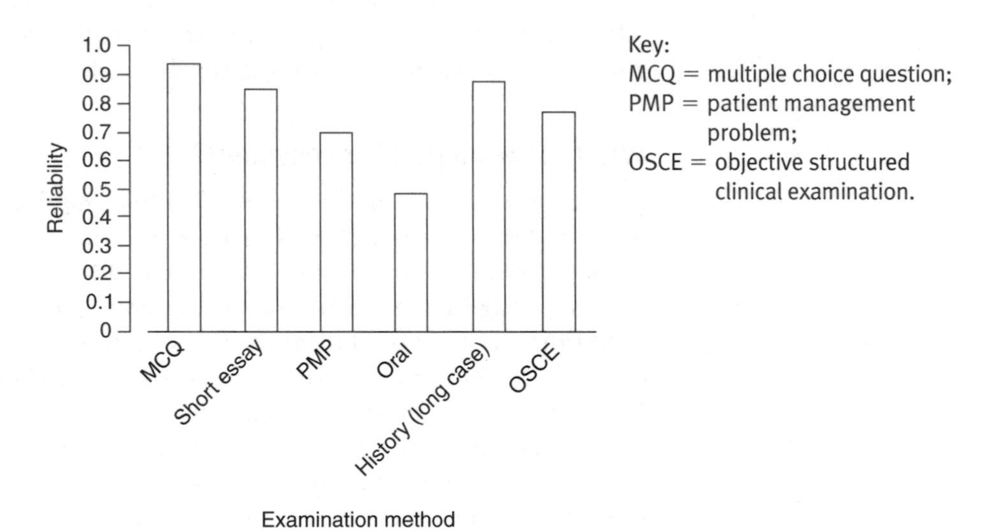

Figure 10.1 Reported reliability when 4 hour testing times are used for different test formats

Of all the subtypes of reliability, the simplest is '**test–retest reliability**'. If a test is reliable there will be a high positive correlation between the results of two administrations of the test. While conceptually simple, it is essential to ensure that items are not remembered between the tests, usually by allowing a time interval to elapse, and ensuring that students do not learn more in the interval. A way of ensuring that students do not remember the items is to change the format of the test but retain the same objectives. This allows the calculation of '**equivalent forms reliability**', but as it involves considerable work, it is rarely done.

More common is '**split half reliability**' which divides the examination into two and correlates the scores for both halves. This is useful for tests with many items and further statistical techniques, such as *Cronbach's Alpha* may be used to look at the internal consistency of the test.

Given the known problems with objectivity, a measure of '**intra-rater reliability**' and '**inter-rater reliability**' may be useful. Intra-rater reliability refers to the consistency of rating by one rater over time, while inter-rater reliability refers to the difference between the 'hawks' and the 'doves'. Correlational statistics are again used.

Determining reliability using statistical techniques is best done in collaboration with an experienced statistician, who may be contacted through a local unit for Medical Education.

Validity

This means that the test measures what you want it to measure. If you want to know whether your students can cannulate a patient, setting a written question on the uses of venous cannulation is not likely to give you an accurate answer. It would thus be an *invalid* test of students skills in cannulation. However it could be a *valid* test of students knowledge about the indications for cannulation. Validity is dependent on both the structure of the assessment and the instructions given to candidates. The assessment needs to cover the whole course that the students have learned, and not concentrate on just one or two areas. The items in the test should be clearly worded, designed to test the outcome (skills, knowledge, or attitudes), and pitched at the right level to discriminate between students. Adequate time needs to be allowed and the students should understand what is expected of them. If all these criteria are fulfilled it is likely that a test is valid.

Factors affecting validity

- **Content.** The test should cover the whole area taught (like reliability, validity is likely to increase with an increase in numbers of items).
- **Structure.** The test needs to be appropriate for the outcome measured (i.e. an MCQ to measure knowledge).
- **Discriminating questions.** Questions should be pitched at the right level to discriminate between candidates (if they are too easy everyone passes).
- **Production.** The items need to be clearly worded (see below).
- **Instructions to candidates.** These need to be clear and unambiguous.
- **Time.** Adequate time needs to be allowed.

Ensuring that an examination is valid requires the following steps.

- Test design: using a '**blueprint**' (see below), selecting the correct format, and planning enough time.
- Question writing: using discriminating questions (see below).
- Proof-reading: to ensure comprehensibility.
- Pre-exam briefing: giving clear instructions to candidates and examiners.

As a marker you are likely to be involved only with the final stage. However you may be asked to write questions, and contribute to developing a 'blueprint'.

Five main types of validity are recognized, all of which contribute to overall validity.

The lay meaning of validity corresponds best to **face validity**. If face validity is high this implies that the exam seems to be appropriate and fair to both teachers and students. Establishing that the exam actually does measure the stated outcomes requires a measurement of **content validity**. This is divided into ***item validity*** and ***sampling validity***. Item validity refers to the appropriateness of the items to the intended outcomes, whereas sampling validity looks at how evenly the questions are spread across the entire course content. In order to ensure content validity the course content and expected outcomes must be accurately known. The next stage is to draw up a '**blueprint**' which lists the expected outcomes on one axis and the content areas tested (i.e. knowledge, problem solving) along the other. This ensures item validity (all questions should fit in on the grid) and sampling validity (number of questions in each area is appropriate, and no areas are missed out).

A small portion of a blueprint from an undergraduate psychiatry assessment is shown below. Blueprints for actual courses will have many more rows and columns. There is a tick for every question that covers a topic—as you can see, some areas have more than one tick, indicating that they were covered by two or more questions. In completing a blueprint you will want to ensure that there is at least one tick in every row and column.

	Knowledge	Application knowledge/ problem solving	History taking	Mental state exam
Psychosis and mania	✓	✓	✓	✓✓
Depression and suicide	✓✓	✓✓	✓✓	
Anxiety, panic disorder somatization, and phobias	✓	✓	✓	
The older patient: acute/chronic confusion	✓✓	✓✓	✓	✓

The degree to which the result of a test relates to future behaviours (e.g. passing finals) is referred to as **predictive validity**. The performance of a new type of test can be correlated with an established test, with a high positive correlation showing good **concurrent validity**. Finally, **construct validity** refers to the degree to which a test correlates to a non-stated outcome, such as patient centredness.

Establishing validity is important as there have been legal challenges in the USA based on invalid assessment design (McManus, 1998, quoted in Fry *et al.*, 1999).

Standards

The traditional method of deciding who passes an exam is to use cut-off points. This might give the top 10% of students an A, the next 40% a B, etc. This is termed

norm-referencing. It is often used within very large cohorts (e.g. all students taking GCSE Maths), as it is reasonable to assume that ability is normally distributed, and does not vary from year to year. However in medical training we are interested in whether a small cohort of students are competent enough to become safe doctors. We can't make this decision by deciding that the bottom 5% are not competent—supposing the entire cohort were poor students: perhaps 30% might not be competent (see graph below).

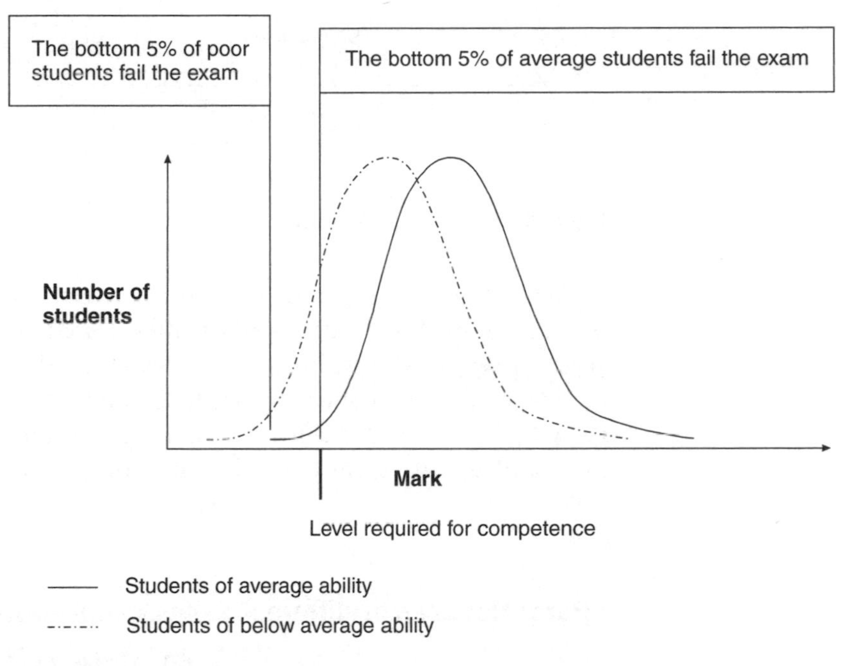

Figure 10.2 Variation of pass mark in norm-referenced test

Getting around this is easy—we simply need to measure the students against a pre-set level of competence, rather then against each other. An example of this is the driving test, which ensures that the learner driver is skilled enough to be safe, and does not depend on who else was tested that day or week. This is termed **criterion referencing** and is commonly used in medical schools today.

Assessment techniques

There are lots of different techniques of assessment, but all have the ultimate aim of assessing whether our students are competent to become doctors. In clinical practice we blend knowledge, skills, and attitudes together to manage our patients. Competence can be divided into levels as shown in the diagram below, devised by Miller (1990). We cannot test our medical students' performance in the 'real world' as they are not yet clinicians. The pragmatic alternative is to focus on the bottom three steps of the pyramid, and assume that if a student reaches the required standard, they will be clinically competent.

Each level can be tested by different assessment techniques. Many assessment techniques are used to assess knowledge and skills. Their use varies slightly between schools. If asked to be a marker, or to advise students on a technique it is a good idea to clarify the type of assessment and the examiner's role with an experienced colleague.

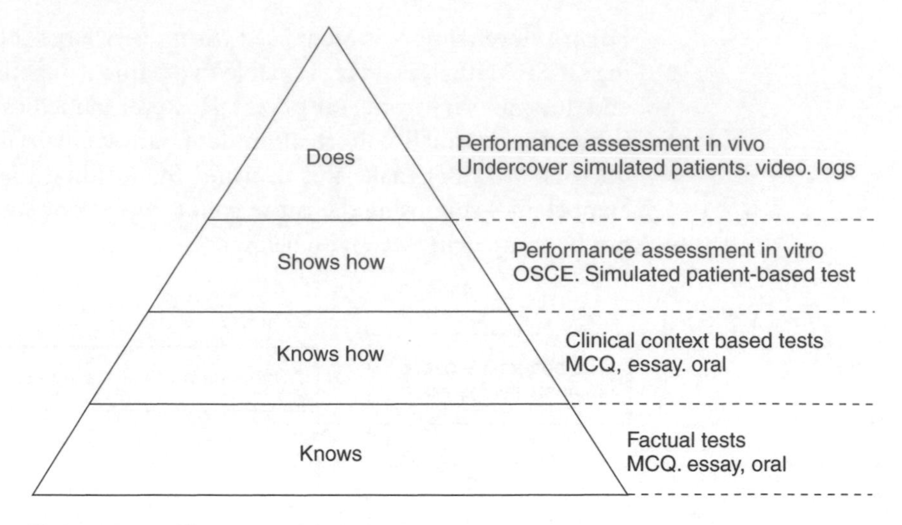

Figure 10.3 Miller's pyramid of competence

The techniques vary in their appropriateness for assessing knowledge, skills, and attitudes. Knowledge is most often tested by written responses (essays, short answers, MCQs, MEQs, and orals). Skills are tested using traditional clinical cases (either short or long), objective structured clinical examinations (OSCEs), and orals for clinical reasoning. Attitudes are rarely assessed in isolation, and usually form part of a question primarily aimed at knowledge or skills.

Potential uses of different assessment tools

	Knowledge	Clinical skills	Other skills*	Attitudes
MCQ (multiple choice questions)	✓			
EMQ (extended matching uestions)	✓			
Short answer questions	✓			
MEQ (modified essay question)	✓		✓	✓
Essays	✓			✓
Projects/dissertations and portfolios	✓		✓	✓
OSCEs (objective structured clinical examinations)	✓	✓	✓	✓
Short and long clinical cases	✓	✓	✓	
End-of-firm assessment	✓	✓	✓	✓
Logbooks		✓		
Presentations	✓		✓	
Orals/vivas	✓		✓	✓

* Other skills including problem solving, communication skills, presentation skills.

The accuracy of all these assessments depends on the quality of the technique used and the objectivity of the examiners.

Getting involved with formal summative assessments

As a medical teacher you may participate in many forms of assessment. When you start teaching, you are most likely get involved in forms of assessment where many markers are needed, such as OSCEs, clinical assessments, and orals. However, while examiners in OSCEs can be relatively inexperienced, those in clinicals and orals should have experience and training to develop objectivity. You may be needed as a marker immediately after the assessment to mark the papers (essays, short answer questions) or help writing MCQs.

Medical students are highly motivated by assessments, and look to their teachers for guidance. Their performance is affected by the quality of the briefing they get, and as a minimum you should be familiar with the organization, technique of assessment, and standards expected.

Key information for briefing students

- **Format**, e.g. OSCE, MCQ.
- **Duration**. How long and how many questions will they have to answer?
- **Organization**. Where, when, any equipment needed (e.g. white coats, stethoscopes, pens/paper).
- **Preparation**. Good techniques include: practice papers for MCQs and short answer papers, timed systems examinations with peer group for OSCEs, clerking and presenting patients to clinical team for clinical examinations.

Techniques for assessing knowledge

The knowledge required of medical practitioners is very large, and to be sure of sampling all the potential content areas, we need to use tools that can rapidly and economically look at breadth of knowledge as well as depth. The tools available can be divided into:

- Objective tests (e.g. MCQs and extended matching questions/EMQs).
- Constructed response tests (e.g. short answer questions).
- Projects and portfolios.
- Orals or vivas.

Of these, portfolios assess skills as well as knowledge. Each of these methods has a different reliability/validity profile.

Reliability/validity profiles in knowledge assessment

	Reliability	Validity	Feasibility
Objective tests	+++	+++	+++
Constructed response	+	++	+
Projects and portfolios	+	++	+
Orals/vivas	+	+	+

Objective tests

All objective tests ask the candidate either to agree or disagree with a statement, or to select one option from a list.

Multiple choice questions (MCQs)

All of us have experienced MCQs. They are probably the most commonly used technique to test knowledge. This is because they are easy to mark (particularly with optically marked answer sheets), and economical of staff time. If well designed, they can sample a large content area, and are reliable due to the high number of questions they contain. Many schools have developed question banks, which reduce the time needed to prepare the exam.

Students often confuse MCQs with multiple true/false questions. Sample questions of both types are shown below.

Sample questions

True/false *circle the correct answer*

Corticosteroid injection improves the symptoms of carpal tunnel syndrome.

T F

MCQ *circle the correct answer*

Carcinoma of the stomach occurs most commonly in:

A Japanese women.

B British men.

C White American men.

D Japanese men.

E Australian women.

In an MCQ, the initial statement is often referred to as the **stem**, and the incorrect answers as the **distractors**. The probability of guessing the correct answer in an MCQ is relatively low (1:5), compared with simple true/false questions, where the probability is1:2.

There are disadvantages to MCQs, in that they do not allow the candidate to display the depth of their knowledge, and it may be difficult to test higher level intellectual skills such as problem solving. Individual items are difficult to write well, and the full exam needs to be carefully constructed with a blueprint (see p. 152) to ensure adequate coverage of the curriculum.

Writing a good MCQ

Stem. Make sure that the detail is clear, avoid irrelevant information, and do not include any negatives. Avoid vague terms like generally, occasionally, and sometimes.

Distractors. Make them all about the same length, grammatically credible, and convincing. Avoid implausible responses, terms such as always or never (the answers are usually false), and vary the position of the correct response in the group.

Grammar. Keep the grammatical structure as simple as possible, avoiding negatives and keeping all responses appropriate to the stem.

Instructions. Keep these short and clear (e.g. circle the correct response).

Piloting. Try questions out on colleagues for comprehensibility and to make sure that it is at the appropriate standard.

Proof-reading. Ensure that you personally review the proofs, as minor mistakes can radically change the sense of a question.

Extended matching questions (EMQs)

Some of the criticisms of MCQs have been met with the development of extended matching questions. A sample is shown below.

Sample EMQ

Topic: The breathless patient.
Response options:

A	Asthma	**F**	Pulmonary embolus
B	Left ventricular failure	**G**	Acute bronchitis
C	Acute haemorrhage	**H**	Pneumothorax
D	Anaemia	**I**	Lobar pneumonia
E	COPD	**J**	Extrinsic allergic alveolitis

Instructions: What is the most likely diagnosis in each of the patients listed below?

1 Mr J is 76 and presents with a gradual onset of SOB, most noticeable when exercising. He also feels tired, has vague lower abdominal pain, and a recent change in bowel habit. His chest is clear on examination.

(***Answer D***)

2 Mrs X is 28. She presents with an acute onset of SOB following a trip to Scotland. She has right-sided pleuritic chest pain. On examination her chest is clear, but her right calf is swollen. Her only medication is the oral contraceptive pill.

(***Answer F***)

3 Miss A is 21 years old. She presents acutely unwell with a three day history of fever, sweats, rigors, cough, and left-sided chest pain. On examination she has a temperature of 40, bronchial breathing, and creps over the left lower lobe.

(***Answer I***)

EMQs adapt very well to the presentation of clinical vignettes, and are widely used to test for the application of knowledge. Writing EMQs can be difficult, and some practical tips are provided below.

Writing a good EMQ

1 **Content**: identify the outcomes you wish to assess and the relevant contexts.

2 **Topics**: label these clearly and concisely.

3 **Response options**: write these first and keep them concise.

4 **Scenarios**: make these short, credible, and ensure that they match the appropriate response.

5 **Piloting**: try questions out on colleagues for comprehensibility.

6 **Proof-reading**: ensure that you personally review the proofs, as minor mistakes can radically change the sense of a question.

For further information see Case and Swanson (1996).

The interpretation of objective tests has been made easy by the development of computer software which generates statistical analyses. These can be used to look at which questions were answered, and the mean and standard deviations of scores. Individual items can be examined for their ability to discriminate between good and poor students, their level of difficulty, and how useful their distractors were (e.g. no one answered E, so it is a poor distractor). Your local medical education unit will be able to provide assistance with interpreting test results, and further information can be found in Newble and Cannon (1994).

Constructed response tests (CRQs)

All constructed response tests (CRQs) allow the candidate to respond to the question in their own words (Davis, 2001). Their advantages are that they allow the candidate to display breadth of knowledge as well as depth, to develop a reasoned argument (which is important in ethics), and display their problem solving skills. CRQs can include clinical scenarios or interpretation of data, and require the use of higher order thinking rather than simple recall of facts.

Disadvantages are clear to anyone who has had to mark 300 illegible scripts. Marking is time-consuming, subjective, and requires some knowledge of the subject. To achieve reliability, marking should be done using a list of key points and some scripts should be double-marked, increasing the staff time needed. While the results from an MCQ can be ready in hours, those of a CRQ usually take days or weeks. To cover the curriculum fully many items are needed which makes these examinations potentially very long.

CRQs can be described according to the stimulus presented and the form of answer required.

Short answer questions

These are likely to be familiar to you. Students are required to respond to a question which may be written, a photograph, X-rays, laboratory results, or a piece from a journal.

A sample with answers is shown below:

> **Short answer question**
>
> **Topic**: Haematology.
>
> **Stimulus**: Haematology report: Full blood count showing microcytic anaemia.
>
> **Question 1** What is this condition called?
> *Microcytic anaemia*
>
> **Question 2** What is the most common cause of this condition?
> *Iron deficiency*
>
> **Question 3** List 3 common symptoms this patient might have.
> *Dyspnoea (SOB, SOBOE), fatigue, palpitations, headache, tinnitus, anorexia*

Longer short answer questions may be used: e.g. 'Write short notes on the cause of bleeding in the third trimester'. This imposes less structure on the students, who are nonetheless encouraged to keep their answer short and succinct.

Short answer questions can be marked 'blind', although this is difficult if the question is in a specialized area. To increase marker reliability, the preferred answers should be provided, with acceptable options as in question 3. The marker then can only accept these answers.

Clinical problems

Many forms of CRQ have attempted to reproduce clinical problem solving. Names used to describe them include Clinical problems, Modified essay questions (MEQ), and Patient management problems (PMP). They aim to test the application of knowledge in clinical settings. In their simplest form they consist of a clinical scenario followed by a number of questions. These can be elaborated, as in the MEQ, to a problem covering several pages, where the patient's problem evolves over time, and which embraces psychological and social aspects of the case. Cases should be selected with care. Common or potentially catastrophic problems are useful, particularly ones that the successful candidate will soon be facing.

Sample clinical problem

Gareth Davies is 35 years old and has been an insulin-dependent diabetic for 20 years. He uses twice daily insulin and measures his blood glucose about twice a week. His busy lifestyle means he often snacks and misses meals.

1 What are the common causes of long-standing IDDM?

2 You discover that Mr Davies's control is suboptimal. What is the evidence for the benefit of regular blood glucose monitoring?

3 You suspect that Mr Davies lifestyle is contributing to his poor control. What other members of the medical team might you involve, and what help could they offer?

4 Mr Davies is bought to A + E cold, confused, and agitated. His blood glucose measurement is unrecordable. How would you initially manage him?

Essays

The use of questions requiring long written answers is becoming less popular. They are still used, particularly in areas where the ability to construct a reasoned argument is a key skill (e.g. ethics). Good questions are not easy to write and it is wise to include instructions about maximum length and the use of references, etc. Using a marking schedule and making it available to students will improve the quality of future essays. Many marking schedules simply provide a list of key factual points. Essay marking is time-consuming, and if this is all you are assessing, it may be more appropriate to use short answer questions. In essays where students are expected to develop a line of argument a focus on the structure and presentation of the essay as well as the content is important. A potential marking schedule, with space for comment is shown overleaf.

Preparing students for a CRQ paper

Encourage students to read the question carefully and note down ideas on a piece of rough paper before starting. They should then structure their work clearly, using headings and underlining where appropriate. They should attempt to keep their writing as legible as possible and use lists or bullet points of important features as they are easier to mark. Finally, students need to be sure that they allow enough time to answer all the questions, as questions are usually evenly weighted.

Essay marking schedule

Student identifier: ______________________ **Date:** __________

Essay title: ______________________

Criteria	Pass	Fail	Mark pass/fail and comments
Major criteria			
Structure	Clear structure: introduction, main discussion, and summary with paragraphs used to contain sections of connected argument.	The student has included neither an introduction nor a summary. The essay is not broken into paragraphs.	
Evidence of reflection	Work shows thought about the topic not just paraphrased other material.	There are no sentences indicating reflection.	
Attitudes expressed	All attitudes the student expresses are appropriate for a health care professional.	Attitudes are expressed that are at odds with the GMCs ethical framework and/or are offensive.	
Breadth of knowledge	Covers more than half of the key points required by question's author.	Less than half of the key points are mentioned.	
Depth of knowledge	More than half of the key points are discussed in depth.	Less than half of the key points have been discussed in any depth (less than one sentence on each point).	
Standard criteria			
Fluency and use of language	Language is appropriate for a university student. Terminology and description is professional and avoids slang. Easy for the reader to understand meaning.	Exceptional number of grammatical errors (sections require re-reading to understand). Frequent use of colloquialism or . inappropriate language	
Focus on the question	The arguments outlined address the question.	The essay question is not addressed at all.	
Coherence/logical argument	Arguments are linked logically, and lead to the conclusions drawn.	Fragmented such that argument cannot be followed. Repeatedly disconnected or contradictorystatements.	
Presentation	Legible font (Arial/ Times roman). Double spaced.	Not word processed.	
Reference to evidence	Any evidence quoted is referenced appropriately.	Includes no references or references are inaccurately quoted. Clear plagi.	
Illustrates arguments with clinical experience	Student shows ability to apply principles to the patients seen on attachment or to include their own experience with patients to illustrate points appropriately.	Fails to include any information from clinical attachment to illustrate arguments. Patient information is disclosed in a way that identifies the patient.	
	Final grade		**Pass/fail comments**

Writing a good constructed response question

1 **Content**: identify the outcomes you wish to assess and the relevant context.

2 **Topics**: label these clearly and concisely.

3 **Information**: if this is a part of the question choose relevant information in an interesting context—e.g. a well written journal article, biochemical results, or a concise clinical problem. If using photographs or graphs, make sure that these will reproduce clearly.

4 **Question**: frame this clearly and concisely. Check the level of difficulty with colleagues.

5 **Marking schedule**: it is helpful to write this in advance, although it may have to be modified once the first scripts have been reviewed. It should be unambiguous. Ensure that the number of marks offered for each piece of information is clear, and allow marks for clarity and use of well-reasoned argument if appropriate.

6 **Proof-reading**: ensure that you personally review the proofs.

Projects, dissertations, and portfolios

Medical schools are increasingly using methods of assessment that can be used to measure learning over time. The results of a project are unlikely to be affected by an 'off' day, or assessment anxiety. They probably offer a truer representation of the student's ability. Undergraduates have often done projects at school, and are likely to encounter longer dissertations if they do an intercalated degree. Portfolios were originally developed as a postgraduate tool for continuing medical education, but medical schools have realized that by starting them as undergraduates, we can emphasize the importance of lifelong learning.

You are likely to come across students who ask you for help with their projects, and you may be asked by your medical school to become a project supervisor.

Projects, dissertations, and portfolios

Common definitions are:

Project: a short piece of research on a particular topic, carried out individually or in a group, and presented in varied formats (e.g. written, presentation, poster).

Dissertation: a longer written report based on personal research, either original work or a literature review.

Portfolio: a collection of information on the learning experienced by the student over a period of time.

Projects

Your students will be covering a wide range of topics using all sorts of techniques to collect information. Projects not only increase student knowledge and skills in specific areas, but also enhance generic competencies, such as data handling, critical thinking, problem solving, presentation skills, team-working, time management, and communication skills. If the project is well constructed it can be highly motivating for students, who may produce outstanding work. However for a project to be successful it needs to be doable. If asked to be a project supervisor, check that the project outline is feasible within the time allowed, and that any financial implications have been recognized. Problems usually arise because the project is ill-defined or over-ambitious.

Marking projects is time-consuming. Try and mark the project against the expected outcomes, and double-mark important projects. Self-assessment and peer assessment (particularly in presentations or posters) is valuable.

Dissertations

You may get involved with student dissertations if you teach students doing an intercalated degree. Dissertations are longer than projects and all students should have an experienced supervisor to help them. If you are asked to be a supervisor for the first time, remember that supervision takes lots of time and energy. You will need to have expertise in the area, and perhaps assistance from an experienced colleague.

Your role includes ensuring that: deadlines are met, the work is clearly presented, the intellectual foundation of the work is credible, and that the conclusions are valid. Fraud and plagiarism are not unknown, and students need to be reminded of the need for ethical approval and that the work must be original.

Marking a dissertation is similar to a project. However, they are high stakes assessments, and due to their length and complexity need careful double-marking by specialists in the appropriate field and external examiners.

Portfolios

Portfolios have not been used for long in undergraduate assessment, and they are used in different ways by different medical schools. A simple portfolio is a collection of course work and evidence of learning experiences. More complex portfolios encourage students to reflect on experiences, list learning objectives, and show evidence of these having been met.

Portfolios are useful because they monitor the progress made by the student, and allow self-expression and creativity. Portfolios with a reflective element are student centred, foster critical thinking, and encourage effective learning habits. If they are continually assessed they allow teachers to detect problems early on, and can offer a valuable insight into student attitudes. Problems with portfolios arise when students are not motivated to keep them. They are also time-consuming and difficult to mark.

Marking a portfolio depends on the form in which it is presented. Ideally you should be able to see the written work in advance, and then interview the student on the content. To increase reliability you will need more than one examiner, and structured marksheets may be used.

Orals/vivas

Most of us have experienced a viva voce examination during training, and may have firm views on their utility. They cause fierce debate within medical education. Their defenders point to their use in assessing all round knowledge and attitudes, while detractors point out their unreliability, suspect content validity, and existence of other, better ways of assessing knowledge and skills.

The traditional viva uses two examiners who can ask the candidate whatever relevant question they like. In an attempt to increase objectivity, attempts have been made to structure vivas.

If asked to examine in a viva it is wise to talk to experienced colleagues first, and if possible, sit in with experienced examiners. Increasing objectivity can be done by using the technique of blueprinting described above to ensure content validity. If doing a clinical viva, it is helpful to use a series of cases and focus questions around these. The aim is to demonstrate both breadth and depth of knowledge. If a candidate is finding the question easy stop them and move on—either to another subject or to probe in greater depth.

Examining a clinical viva

- **Method**: talk to colleagues and sit in on a viva—this will help you to calibrate your questions and clarify the standard expected of students.
- **Content**: use a blueprint to determine content and devise cases to cover the various areas (e.g. a case about a 14 year old seeking contraception could cover gynae, ethics, and communication skills).
- **Set the scene**: introduce yourself and your fellow examiner and explain the exam format.
- **Technique**: cover ground as efficiently as possible. If a candidate evidently knows the answer, stop them and move on. Change examiners at the half-way point.
- **Record keeping**: keep clear notes of the areas covered and how the student performed.

Techniques for assessing skills

You are likely to come across the following techniques for assessing skills:

- OSCEs
- Clinical long and short cases
- Tutor assessments (end-of-firm reports)
- Logbooks
- Clinical presentations

Assessing a students clinical skills requires observation of the student to detect whether the technique they are using is appropriate and feedback from the student about any abnormalities detected. We often then assess clinical reasoning by asking the students to attempt a differential diagnosis. OSCEs have become popular because they can expose students to a wider number of cases, are relatively objective, and thus seen to be fairer than long or short clinical cases.

All techniques for assessing skills cover some knowledge domains as well. The degree to which the knowledge and skills component can be separated (particularly in the last two forms of assessment) depends on the way the assessment is set up. Each of these methods has a different reliability/validity profile as usually performed.

Reliability/validity profiles in skills assessment

	Reliability	Validity	Feasibility
OSCEs	+++*	+++	+
Clinical cases	+*	+*	++
Tutor assessments	+	++	+++
Logbooks	+	+++	+++
Clinical presentations	+	+	++

* Depends on the number of cases in the examination.

Objective structured clinical examinations (OSCEs)

An OSCE consists of several 'stations', each lasting 5–15 minutes and arranged in a circuit. Students complete each station within the time limit and then move on to the next. To be reliable, a summative OSCE covering a wide curriculum needs over 20 stations, and should take at least $2\frac{1}{2}$ hours.

Each station will have some candidate instructions, an activity (which could involve interviewing or examining a standardized patient, performing a simple test, interpreting a photograph or X-ray, etc.) and a standardized marksheet. Any activity that involves a patient will have a marker present to complete the marksheet.

Sample instruction and marksheets for a short and basic station are shown below.

OSCE Candidates instructions

Station X: Cranial nerves

Mr Smith is a 22-year-old student, who has complained of vague headaches and bumping into things from time to time. This has persisted for 'some time' but seems to be getting worse.

Please examine cranial nerves II, III, IV, and VI. Comment on what you are doing and your findings to the examiner.

OSCE Marksheet

Name________________

Station No: Cranial nerves

Examiner: Please ring one response for each item.

	Done	Not done
General approach to patient	1	0
Comments on appearance of eyes (normal)	1	0
Examines visual acuity (Snellen chart)	1	0
Examines visual fields by confrontation	1	0
Examines external ocular movements	1	0
Asks about diplopia	1	0
Examines pupil response to light	1	0
Examines pupil response to accommodation	1	0
Examines fundi	1	0
Correctly diagnoses bitemporal hemianopia	1	0
TOTAL	**/10**	

OSCEs are considered to be more objective than other forms of clinical assessment. This is due to:

- The marksheet. This limits markers by only allowing them to indicate if a student has or has not performed a certain activity.

- Standardized patients. These are actors or members of the public who had special training to simulate clinical scenarios for students.
- Large number of items. This allows good coverage of the course, and, with a blueprint, reduces possible sampling errors.

Well designed OSCEs are generally seen by students and teachers to be fair. However, there are disadvantages to an OSCE. They are expensive and time-consuming, requiring big halls, lots of equipment, and plenty of markers. It is difficult to re-run OSCEs for students who are absent, and late arrivals or re-sits may pose a problem.

Marking an OSCE

If asked to be a marker, make sure you arrive well before the actual start time to find your station and familiarize yourself with the marksheet. This is particularly important in stations which require you to observe the candidate closely. Check that all the equipment students may need is present, and that you have enough marksheets. Introduce yourself to the simulated patient when they arrive, and make sure that they are familiar with the role that they are to play. It is a good idea to check with the organizers how much prompting of the students is allowed.

Even with a marksheet, markers need to understand what standard the students are expected to reach—was that a good enough assessment of visual fields? When listening to a history-based station it is vital to listen to what the patient says as well as the questions actually asked by the student. This is because standardized patients are usually trained to reveal more to active listeners asking open questions than to students employing repetitive closed questions.

OSCEs often take over two hours per circuit, and are repetitive. They are surprisingly tiring. If facing a full day of examining, choose a comfortable chair and make sure refreshments are available.

Preparing students for an OSCE

It is helpful for students to know how many stations there are and to understand the sort of questions that can be asked. The medical school may offer sample questions. There are now several good OSCE books available for students with sample questions and marking schedules. These are designed to help them understand the format, learn appropriate skills, and perform to the required standard. It can be helpful for students to devise problems for each other and develop marksheets. A blank marksheet is attached for your use. You can help them prepare by letting them see plenty of patients and running through systems examinations with them within a time limit—e.g. perform a knee examination in five minutes.

Students should check what equipment they should take with them. Remind them to read the question carefully and reflect before they start. Encourage them to ask the examiner for clarification if they are unclear about the wording of the question and then talk through what they are doing if appropriate.

Setting an OSCE

Organizing an OSCE is a major undertaking and should be never done without adequate academic and administrative support. If you think that your course would benefit from using an OSCE, speak to your medical education unit, experienced colleagues, and the medical school to ensure adequate funding. For further information see the references at the end of the chapter.

Blank OSCE marksheet

Name of candidate______________________

Name of marker______________________

Problem ____

(e.g. Mr X has had a painful knee after a fall, please examine his knees and comment on your findings.)

Objective *(e.g. Observes both knees, comments on abnormalities.)*	**Done**	**Not done**
	1	0
	1	0
	1	0
	1	0
	1	0
	1	0
	1	0
	1	0
	1	0
	1	0
	1	0
	1	0
Total		

Long and short clinical cases

You are likely to remember these from your own days as a student. In a long case, the student and the patient are left for a period of time, during which the student takes a history and examines the patient. The student then presents the patient to the examiners who examine him or her on features of the case, sometimes returning to the patient to go through aspects of the examination. In short cases the interaction with the patient is much shorter, often limited to a 'spot' diagnosis, or demonstrating a skill, and any questions are also brief.

Clinical cases are perceived to be a valid way to assess clinical competence, although they have many shortcomings (Wilson *et al.*, 1969). This is due to the fact that no two students see the same cases, it is difficult to ensure that the cases cover the course, and inter-rater reliability is low. Increasing reliability and validity depends on increasing the number of cases seen, and the number of examiners rating the student (Wass and Jolly, 2001). However, as they are still used extensively in final examinations, it is important to be as objective as possible.

Marking a clinical long case

If you are asked to mark a clinical examination it helps to get to know the patient first. If possible introduce yourself, check the salient features of the history, and assure yourself that the clinical signs (if any) are still present. The patient's notes are also often available, and there may be a précis of the history. You can increase your objectivity by devising a series of questions that cover the range of the patients complaints, the underlying pathophysiology, and appropriate management. Try and cover as much ground as possible, and include problem solving questions (e.g. 'If this patient then developed haematuria what would you do?'). Once the student has presented the case (which can be rated for accuracy and clarity) prompt them to attempt a differential diagnosis. You can then run through your questions, moving on as soon as it is clear that the student is familiar with the ground, and score them on their performance. The reliability of long cases is increased if students are observed and their performance rated using a checklist, but this is not current practice in most medical schools (Feather and Fry, 1999).

Marking short cases

In short cases the student will go from patient to patient. It is again helpful to familiarize yourself with the cases and check signs beforehand. In order to increase objectivity, select up to six patients (depending on the total number of patients and the time available) who have varied problems, and devise questions on each patient. You can then see the patients in the same order with each of the students.

Preparing students for clinical cases

It is helpful for students to have plenty of clerking and presentation practice. You may be able to identify patients, listen to presentations, or hold practice examinations. It is helpful for students to experience the sort of questions that they are likely to be asked following their presentation, and this can be incorporated into ward rounds or clinical tutorials.

Tutor assessments

Many courses and attachments will have a tutor assessment at the end. These vary across courses and across medical schools, from a bald '*clinical firm 2–B*' to detailed structured reports, looking at a student's performance in various areas. These assessments are important as they can provide a view of the student's performance over time. The student's performance in the clinical setting can be assessed together with other attributes which are difficult to assess by other methods. These include generic competencies such as team-work and time management, personal attributes and attitudes. There is no doubt that tutor assessments are very useful, particularly for providing references for students as they move into their PRHO year, or for probing the performance of problem students.

However there are problems with end-of-firm reports. It is common to hear students complain:

'X and I both got a B, despite the fact that X was never there.'

'I got a C from the Prof, just because I made a mess of one case on the first ward round.'

'You have to be fantastic on the cardio firm to get an A whereas half of the renal firm got an A, and the rest got Bs.'

Using structured forms, and asking more then one teacher to complete the form can address this lack of reliability and objectivity.

Completing a tutor assessment

If you have been provided with a structured form, it is helpful to have a look at it before the rotation starts, so that you can be sure of collecting the appropriate information. If a form is not provided it is wise to discuss the areas you will be expected to assess with colleagues. In the clinical setting it is likely that you will be expected to grade and comment on the following areas:

(a) Clinical skills.

(b) Generic competencies: communication skills, relationship with patients and with the health care team, reliability.

(c) Personal attributes: attendance, dress and appearance, attitude towards patients, interest and motivation.

A sample structured form for a clinical attachment is provided opposite.

Doing end-of-attachment reports often seems like a thankless task. It is helpful to set aside time to do them, and ensure that you have enough information on each student to fill them in accurately. It is very helpful for the student and medical school to add your own comments alongside the grades. On large firms it may be difficult to recall the student, and talking to other members of staff is helpful.

In some cases the report may be filled in with the student present, and this is a valuable time for detailed feedback on their performance. It is often helpful to ask the students what they feel they did well, and not so well on the firm as a way of starting the interview, and using the structure of the form to help students understand what is expected of them.

Logbooks

Logbooks are used by many medical schools to monitor students' acquisition of skills. They are usually used formatively, and you may have to review a students logbook as part of a tutor assessment. Logbooks usually contain a list of the skills that the students should encounter, and are often subdivided into skills the student should be able to do and skills they should witness. Students may ask you to witness them performing a skill in order to 'sign it off'. To do this properly needs close observation, and you will also be able to give the student valuable feedback. Logbooks may contain lists of conditions that the students should encounter, and you may be asked for help in finding appropriate patients.

Logbooks are a type of portfolio, but concentrate on skills rather than the global learning. Because they are designed to be portable they are a useful aide memoire for students, and help to ensure coverage of the curriculum.

End-of-firm assessment

Name:_______________ **Date:**_______________

Firm/specialty_______________

Hospital_______________ **Assessor**_______________

Please use the guidelines below to assess students performance in the following areas, and then award a final OVERALL grade.

Knowledge	A	B	C	D
History taking	A	B	C	D
Clinical skills	A	B	C	D
Communication skills	A	B	C	D
Attitude	A	B	C	D
Attendance	Satisfactory/unsatisfactory			
Overall grade	A	B	C	D

What went well?

What could you/they do better?

	A	B	C	D
Knowledge	Excellent.	Very good.	Satisfactory.	Weak.
History taking	Excellent.	Good.	Acceptable.	Unacceptable.
Clinical skills	Able to carry out a wide range of skills to an excellent standard.	Able to carry out a range of skills to a good standard.	Able to carry out some skills to an acceptable standard.	Unable to carry out skills to the required standard.
Communication skills	Communicates very well, always using appropriate verbal and non-verbal skills.	Communicates well, mostly using appropriate skills.	Acceptable communication skills.	Unacceptable communication skills.
Attitude	Excellent attitude, treated staff, patients, tutor, and colleagues at all times with respect.	Good attitude and professional approach.	Acceptable attitude to staff patients, tutor, and colleagues.	Demonstrated poor attitude: concerns re development of a professional approach.
Overall grade	The top 10% of students may achieve this.	The top 25% of the year may achieve this.	The majority of students.	The students progress should be reviewed by the sub-dean.

Unfortunately students often don't fill them in unless encouraged, and the lack of a reflective component in the majority of logbooks means that they don't actively encourage lifelong learning.

When assessing a logbook it is useful to go over it with the student. The way in which it has been filled in and their insights into the further learning needed may give you information on their attitudes.

Presentations

Presentations are being increasingly used for assessment. Many schools provide audio-visual aids for student use, and student presentations are often very professional. Presentations can be patient based, reflect project work, or focus on a particular topic area. If the student can choose their subject it is helpful to check that it is appropriate before they start work. Presentations are motivating for students, and provide a good insight into a student's understanding of the subject. If students work together on a presentation, it is possible to assess team-work, but the composition of the group and the different contributions of each group member have to be taken into account. Drawbacks of presentations are that they are time-consuming to mark, and depend heavily on the student's individual presentation skills.

Presentations can be marked by both the teacher and the other students in the audience. Once again, objectivity is increased by the use of an assessment instrument, and a sample is included opposite.

Assessing attitudes

Medical schools have developed attitudinal objectives (General Medical Council, 1993) but are often not assessing students on them. This may reflect the fact that attitudes are difficult to assess because they cannot be measured directly. Attitudes can only be inferred through the way in which a student behaves, either in the clinical situation, or in answer to a questionnaire. The three ways that have been used to assess attitudes are:

- Direct self-report questionnaires
- Paper cases
- Observation of behaviour

Assessing attitudes is made harder by the fact that students will give the answer that they think the medical school wants to hear. This 'response bias' may only be overcome if a student feels very strongly about an issue.

Questionnaires

These are reliable, cheap (once they have been developed), and easy to administer. They ask students how they *think* they would behave in a given set of circumstances, but because they don't place students in an actual clinical situation they are a poor guide to actual behaviour. Even where responses are anonymized, they are prone to response bias.

Paper cases

These start with a description of a case (either written or in video format), followed by questions on the actions the student might take. Using clinical scenarios makes them more clinically relevant, and gives them greater validity than questionnaires. However they probably suffer similar response biases. While they simulate a real situation, they are no substitute for observing what a student does in practice.

Assessment of presentation

Date:____________________ **Title:**____________________

Presenters name(s):____

Criteria for assessment	**Grade**
Preparation: done background work, know what they are talking about.	....
Clarity: of speech and materials used. Understandable, not overloaded with facts.	....
Structured: beginning/middle/end, clear objectives, good summary, clear signposting of different stages.	....
Pace: well paced (not too fast/slow, finish on time).	....
Interesting: use different media (e.g. flip chart, OHP, talking, questions), change presenters (when appropriate).	....
Interactive: talk to the audience/eye contact, involve audience (e.g. using questions), tone of voice (interested/enthusiastic).	....

What went well?

What could you/they do better?

Grading system: 1 = Poor. 2 = Fair. 3 = Average. 4 = Good. 5 = Excellent

Overall grade /5

Assessing attitudes is far from straightforward, and very few schools attempt a systematic approach to it, let alone one based on an assessment strategy that is both reliable and valid.

Several instruments have been developed. De Monchy's Doctor–Patient scale (de Monchy *et al.*, 1988; Markert, 1989) is a questionnaire which attempts to discriminate between students who are doctor centred/disease orientated and those who are patient centred/problem orientated. The Professional Decisions and Values Test (PDV) (Rezler *et al.*, 1992), is a formative, diagnostic test, uses written case vignettes to assess students underlying values in situations of ethical uncertainty.

Observation has high validity, but the reliability depends on several factors. Studies of the behaviour of junior doctors have been carried out using nursing staff, senior medical staff, and patients (Woolliscroft *et al.*, 1994; Klessig *et al.*,) as observers. Opinions of patients and staff members often do not correlate (Klessig *et al.*,), suggesting either they are assessing differing aspects, or that doctors behaviour changes in the presence of their seniors, an example of a possible response bias. This problem with reliability might be overcome by clearly specifying target behaviours, staff training, and a large sampling frame (at least 50 patient observations per doctor) (Woolliscroft *et al.*, 1994). Observation has already been used formatively (Papadakis *et al.*, 1999), in the USA. Another approach is to use simulated patients (Rezler, 1976) within an OSCE (Cohen *et al.*, 1991), acknowledging that this reduces validity and increases the potential for response bias.

Observation

This looks at the student's behaviour in practice and, in the form of a tutors report, has been used for a long time. While it remains the most valid approach, it is time-consuming, and has poor inter-rater reliability. An alternative is to use simulated patients and increase objectivity using trained observers (for example in an OSCE examination). This method is still being developed, but seems quite promising, and you may encounter it as part of summative assessments.

Assessing attitudes is not straightforward. Self-report questionnaires, paper cases, and observations of behaviour all have benefits but important limitations (as summarized below). You may have to combine all three to assess your students attitudes in a reliable, valid, and feasible way.

Reliability/validity in attitudinal assessment

	Reliability	Validity	Feasibility
Direct self-report questionnaires	+++	+	+++
Paper cases	++	++	+++
Observation of behaviour	+	+	+
Use of simulated patients	++	++	++

Designing an assessment

Assessments have different purposes and come in different sizes. It may be easy to set a formative test for the students you have recently been teaching, but putting together a large summative examination is a difficult task. If asked to become involved it is wise to set up a team to help you. The team might include other teachers in your subject area who have prior experience of examinations, help from your medical education unit, and administrative support.

The initial step will be developing a blueprint with your team to help you to cover all the ground fairly. The type of assessment technique you select depends on the outcomes you wish to assess, and is often a balance between 'best' and 'feasible'. Once it has been determined you can set the date and time of the examination (this should be done well in advance as large rooms can be hard to book).

If you are using a written exam you may already have a bank of questions to call on, but otherwise you will need to write the questions with your team. Ensure that model answers are also written, and that tight security is maintained. Proof-read all final drafts yourself, and get a colleague to check them for any mistakes you might miss. A team of markers should be in place to mark (and possibly double-mark) the scripts after the exam, unless you have used a format that can be automatically marked using optical scanning techniques. It is good practice to have a meeting with the markers beforehand to fully brief them about the examination. Once the examination is over you will need to distribute the scripts to your markers. It may be possible to get the markers together to mark, and this should increase objectivity, as difficult cases can be immediately discussed. After marking, you will need to collect the scripts back and collate the marks.

If you plan a clinical examination, you may also have a bank of questions to call on if you have chosen an OSCE format. If you are using a short/long case clinical exam you will need to recruit patients. In both cases you will need to find appropriate accommodation and recruit and train markers. You will need to ensure that appropriate equipment and paperwork is prepared, and that you have a system for the collation and distribution of marks.

Practical assessment tips

1 Design your course with clear objectives as this will make assessment easier.
2 Assemble an assessment team of teachers, educationalists, and administrators.
3 Choose an appropriate assessment technique.
4 Use a 'blueprint' to ensure that you have covered the curriculum.
5 Ensure that you have the resources (man-power, materials, space, money) required.
6 Fully brief and train examiners.
7 Brief students.
8 Collate marks and disseminate, with appropriate feedback.

Conclusion

Assessing students is a difficult task. Assessment is made easier if your course has clear objectives or outcomes against which the students can be tested. To ensure that an assessment is accurate, it needs to be reliable and valid. To be reliable a test needs to be objective, while to be valid it needs to cover the whole course fairly. When designing an assessment, you will want to choose the best technique you can and this will depend on the outcomes you want to assess, and the resources you have available.

Each medical school uses several assessment techniques to cover the whole field of medicine. Some tests are designed to be more objective than others, and as an examiner you need to take this into account. Designing an assessment is challenging, and is best done by a team of teachers with help from your medical education unit.

References

Ausubel, D. P., Novak, J. S., and Hanesian, H. (1978) *Educational psychology: a cognitive view*, 2nd edn. New York: Holt, Rinehart and Winston.

Case, S. M., and Swanson, D. B. (1996) *Constructing written test questions for the basic and clinical sciences*. Philadelphia: National Board of Examiners.

Cohen, R., Singer, P. A., Rothman, A. I., and Robb, A. (1991) Assessing competency to address ethical issues in medicine. *Acad Med* **66**, 14–5.

Curzon, L. B. (1994) Teaching in further education: an outline of principles and practice, 4th edn. London: Cassell Education.

Davis, M. (2001) Constructed response questions. In *A practical guide for medical teachers* (ed. J. A. Dent and R. Harden), pp. 326–35. Edinburgh: Churchill Livingstone.

de Monchy, C., Richardson, R., Brown, R. A., and Harden, R. M. (1988) Measuring attitudes of doctors: the doctor-patient (DP) rating. *Med Educ* **22**, 231–9.

Dent, J. A., and Harden, R. (ed.) (2001) *A practical guide for medical teachers*. Edinburgh: Churchill Livingstone.

Feather, A., and Fry, H. (1999) Key aspects of teaching and learning in medicine and dentistry. In *A handbook for teaching and learning in higher education: enhancing academic practice* (ed. H. Fry, S. Ketteridge, and S. Marshall). London: Kogan Page.

Fry, H., Ketteridge, S., and Marshall, S. (ed.) (1999) *A handbook for teaching and learning in higher education: enhancing academic practice*. London: Kogan Page.

General Medical Council. (1993) *Tomorrow's doctors. Recommendations on undergraduate medical education*. General Medical Council, London.

Guilford, J. P. (1974) *Psychometric methods*, 2nd edn. New York: McGraw-Hill.

Klessig, J., Robbins, A. S., Wieland, D., and Rubenstein, L. (1989) Evaluating humanistic attributes of internal medicine residents. *J Gen Intern Med* **4**, 514–21.

Markert, R. J. (1989) Cross-cultural validation of the Doctor–Patient Scale. *Acad Med* **64**, 690.

Miller, G. E. (1990) The assessment of clinical skills/competence/performance. *Acad Med* **65**, 563–7.

Newble, D., and Cannon, R. (1994) *A handbook for medical teachers*, 3rd edn. London: Kluwer Academic Publishers.

Papadakis, M. A., Osborn, E. H., Cooke, M., and Healy, K. (1999) A strategy for the detection and evaluation of unprofessional behavior in medical students. University of California, San Francisco School of Medicine Clinical Clerkships Operation Committee. *Acad Med* **74**, 980–90.

Rezler, A. G. (1976) Methods of attitude assessment for medical teachers. *Med Educ* **10**, 43–51.

Rezler, A. G., Schwartz, R. L., Obenshain, S. S., Lambert, P., Gibson, J. M., and Bennahum, D. A. (1992) Assessment of ethical decisions and values. *Med Educ* **26**, 7–16.

Rowntree, D. (1977) *Assessing students*. London: Harper and Row.

Wass, V., and Jolly, B. (2001) Does observation add to the validity of the long case? *Med Educ* **35**, 729–34.

Wass, V., van der Vleuten, C., Shatzer, J., and Jones, R. (2001) Assessment of clinical competence. *Lancet* **357**, 945–9.

Wilson, G. M., Level, R., Harden, R. M., Robertson, J. B., and MacRitchie, J. (1969) Examination of clinical examiners. *Lancet* **1**, 37–40.

Woolliscroft, J. O., Howell, J. D., Patel, B. P., and Swanson, D. B. (1994) Resident–patient interactions: the humanistic qualities of internal medicine residents assessed by patients, attending physicians, program supervisors, and nurses. *Acad Med* **69**, 216–24.

Further reading

Case, S. M., and Swanson, D. B. (1996) *Constructing written test questions for the basic and clinical sciences.* Philadelphia: National Board of Examiners.

Dent, J. A., and Harden, R. (ed.) (2001) *A practical guide for medical teachers.* Edinburgh: Churchill Livingstone.

Rowntree, D. (1977) *Assessing students.* London: Harper and Row.

Acknowledgement

We are grateful for the input of Dr. Jonathan Martin MMedSci (Clin Ed), MRCGP, ILTM, Senior Teaching Fellow, Royal Free and University College Medical School, London, with the writing of this chapter.

CHAPTER 11
Evaluating teaching and learning

After extensive preparation, and using your wide range of teaching skills, you have delivered what you consider to be several excellent teaching sessions. The students seemed happy enough, and you felt pleased afterwards. Still, you have some doubts. As a reflective teacher, you ask yourself how good they really were.

To find out how good the sessions were means asking yourself whether they helped the students learn. Asking the students and looking at their assessment results are the most direct way of finding out, but you will also have views and so will other teachers on your course. Collecting information from all these people is only useful if you can use it to improve your teaching. The information you collect needs to be sufficiently specific to tell you what needs attention. Getting the right information from the right sources is the key to a useful evaluation.

Every session is part of a course, and you may go on to ask yourself whether your session was a valuable part of the course, and whether the course was useful. Evaluating teaching can be done at an individual, course, departmental, or institutional level. This chapter looks at what evaluation of teaching means, why and how all teachers should evaluate teaching, and what to do following a poor evaluation.

What is evaluation?

Many people find the terms 'evaluation' and 'assessment' confusing in an educational context. As discussed in Chapter 10, evaluation measures the *quality* of teaching, either at an individual, course, or institutional level, while assessment measures how much the learner has learned. We all continuously evaluate teaching sessions and respond to feedback from our students by altering the pace or content of the session. After teaching, most of us will have a feeling about how successful the session was. This may be an accurate or a wholly inaccurate assessment of what actually happened. This chapter will help you to analyse these reflections in more depth, and to seek further information from students and colleagues on the quality of your teaching.

Why evaluate teaching?

From a personal point of view, there are a lot of reasons for teachers to take part in teaching evaluations. Most of us like to know how we have performed and it is very rewarding to receive positive evaluations. If they are detailed enough they can tell you exactly how you can improve your teaching. Not only do they help you develop your teaching skills, but also you can use them as part of a teaching portfolio (see Chapter 12) which may be needed for accreditation or promotion. Evidence of teaching evaluation at course, departmental, and institutional level is required by the Teaching Quality Assurance (TQA) procedures and is useful is you want to apply to a membership organization such as the Institute for Learning and Teaching (ILT). The bottom line is that evaluating teaching has become a core requirement and is something that every teacher will now have to participate in.

What is behind this trend to evaluate teaching? Medical educators, like clinicians, are becoming increasingly accountable for their work. This seems to reflect both a general move towards greater accountability and also pressure for high quality health service from society as a whole. A good health service needs well trained doctors, which in turn leads to investment in teaching. This teaching is expensive, and governments want to be sure that it offers value for money. Finally, changes in the funding of education mean that students are increasingly paying directly for it and they are vociferous in their demands for high quality teaching. As a result, evaluating teaching has a higher profile than ever before.

Evaluation has different purposes, and these critically affect the way in which teachers approach it. The model below (Ramsden, 1992) places the process of evaluation on two dimensions.

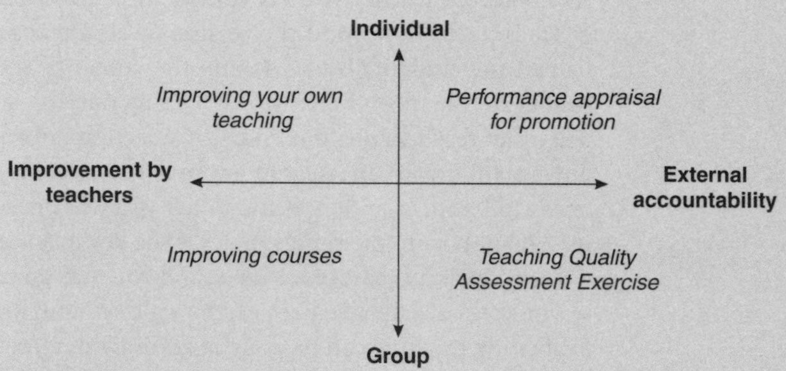

Figure 11.1 Two dimensions of the process of evaluation

Different stakeholders have different interests in the results of an evaluation—for example a teacher may be interested in whether they are assessing prior knowledge adequately; an academic department in whether a teacher merits promotion; an institution in whether teaching load is adversely affecting the research output of the department; and a government official in whether a new programme seems to address current political imperatives (Snell *et al.*, 2000). These different approaches can be regarded as formative and summative, but a well designed evaluation tool should produce data that is appropriate for both purposes.

Principles of evaluation

Evaluation, like assessment, has some basic principles that need to be followed if the results of the evaluation are to be accurate. First, the evaluation tools need to be accurate—and this means that they need to be reliable and valid (see Chapter 10). Using pre-tested evaluation tools, objective and subjective approaches, and multiple sources of information will increase both reliability and validity. Secondly, the information that you gather needs to be useful. This is more likely if you have used a combination of quantitative and qualitative techniques. Thirdly, the evaluation needs to be feasible. If it is too burdensome or not acceptable to teachers or those who have to complete it, it will not be used at all.

It is tempting to think that every time a session or course goes wrong, there is a problem with the teaching. To make sure that the success or failure of a course is put in context, you need to collect information about the input into the course (for example abilities of the students, design and planning of the course), process (the way in which the course was administered, taught, and assessed), and the outcomes of the course (Newble and Cannon, 1994).

A teaching programme can be assessed at different levels as shown below. The higher the level, or the more complicated the new programme, the more complicated it is to assess.

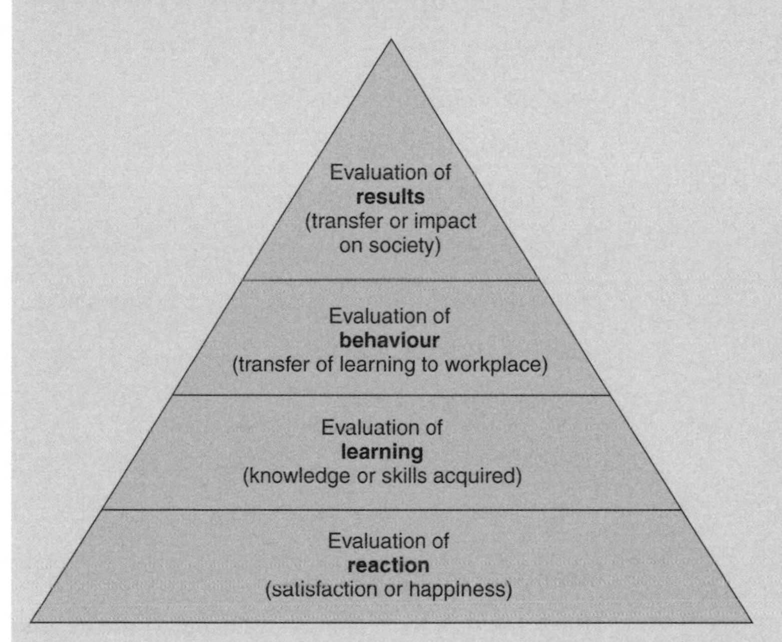

Kirkpatrick's hierarchy of levels of evaluation (Kirkpatrick 1967)

Low level evaluations may be very useful for planning improvements to a course, and may be informative to a wide audience when published. To really assess whether new teaching techniques produce better doctors, we need to evaluate effects further up the pyramid. This is complex and expensive, and needs long-term follow-up of students. For their results to be accurate, evaluations need to use rigorous standards of reliability and validity in both quantitative and qualitative methodologies. This requires gathering information from multiple sources—'triangulation'—using reliable instruments (Rippey, 1981). The boundaries between evaluations and research are blurred—in that many evaluations are published (Wilkes and Bligh, 1999) and treated as if they were research. However, unless they adhere to high scientific standards, they cannot be considered to be research.

Evaluating your teaching session

Depending on whether the evaluation is for personal, course, or institutional reasons, your approach will vary. The methods you use for individual self-evaluation for your own personal development may be different from those required by external assessment processes for your institution as a whole. In this chapter we will consider approaches to evaluation at individual and course levels. We have not addressed departmental or institutional evaluation in detail in this chapter as these are of less direct relevance to the individual teacher and are better investigated in a more specialized texts (Dent and Harden, 2001; Rippey, 1981).

There are a number of steps you can take to evaluate your own teaching, ranging from simple things that could be introduced immediately through to more complex activities for which you may require some external support. These have been summarized below.

Methods for evaluating your teaching session

Attendance figures.

Student evaluation forms.

Informal self-reflection.

Structured reflective exercise.

Student performance in assessments.

Your own performance in teaching assessments.

Peer observation or review.

Mentoring.

Appraisal.

Attendance records

This is the simplest method—unhappy students vote with their feet. They boycott teaching sessions if the teaching appears unattractive or irrelevant to them from the pre-course material, title, or their colleagues remarks. It is worth noting how many students select your course or clinical firm, or attend your lecture when they have been given a choice. Obviously many factors will affect attendance levels and a full lecture theatre does not imply good teaching or vice versa.

Informal self-reflection during a session

We all continuously evaluate sessions while we are teaching, and alter our teaching as appropriate. Good teachers are responsive to feedback (verbal and non-verbal cues) from students as a session progresses. Do they look bored and distracted or engaged and interested? Do they understand the key points and can they answer your questions correctly? Are you on target to meet the session objectives?

Informal self-reflection after a session

Many teachers instinctively reflect immediately after a teaching session, although it may often be limited to a transient awareness of a sense of satisfaction or frustration. It is worthwhile spending a few moments considering what happened in the session in a little more detail. For example you can ask yourself what factors made the session go well, and what aspects to the session the students seem to engage with and learn from. You should also reflect on what went poorly, why that might have been and if there is anything you should change for the next time you teach. If you are likely to teach the same session again you can note these points on the back of your teaching plan for future reference.

Structured reflective exercise

It is well worth the additional small effort to put some of your informal reflective thoughts down on paper after the session in a more structured way. This has a number of potential uses. It encourages you to consider and reinforce positive aspects of your teaching (most people find this much more difficult to do than self-criticism), it provides a record which you can refer to in the future, and it can be included as part of a teaching portfolio (see Chapter 12). The form should be completed using the principles of effective feedback, i.e.

(a) Be completed as close as possible to the event.

(b) Contain specific rather than general comments.

(c) Be constructive.

(d) Comment on behaviours you can change rather than personality attributes that are unchangeable.

The content of the form should be tailored to meet your own personal needs and situation, but is likely to include some fairly generic components to any teaching encounter. If you have used a teaching plan, use the reflection form on the back. Otherwise the form shown overleaf may be helpful. The quantitative section will enable you to focus on different parts of the session, while the qualitative section helps you to look in depth at the quality of your teaching.

Student performance in assessments

While it is clear that student performance in assessments directly relates to their learning, it is easy to forget that this also relates at least in part to your teaching and can be used for the purposes of teaching evaluation. You could use both formal student assessments (such as examination results) and more informal assessments that you have integrated into the session itself to contribute to the evaluation of your teaching.

Student evaluation forms

Forms completed by the students at the end of the session or course are the commonest formal method of evaluation. The quality of feedback you receive will relate directly to the style and content of the evaluation form itself. Good evaluation forms will usually include a mixture of closed quantitative questions and open more qualitative questions. The 'closed' questions usually include rating some aspect of your teaching on a scale of 1 to 5 which is good for comparing your performance over time or against your peers but lacks depth and does not give insights into how you can improve things. The 'open' questions often ask what went well or badly in the sessions or firm and should encourage specific constructive comments by the students. The box below gives practical tips on designing good evaluation forms for students, with a sample 'generic' student evaluation form. This could be adapted for use in almost any teaching scenario.

Teaching self-assessment form

Subject: ______________________________

Date: ______________________________

Reflecting on your teaching and students learning will make you a better teacher. Spend a few moments completing this form as soon as possible after teaching, and put it in your 'Teaching Portfolio'.

Rate the following:

		Poorly			Effectively
Intro:	Motivated students	1	2	3	4
	Assessed learners needs/knowledge	1	2	3	4
	Agreed aims and objectives	1	2	3	4
Body:	Set pace at right level	1	2	3	4
	Set level of difficulty	1	2	3	4
	Promoted student interaction	1	2	3	4
	Assessed student learning	1	2	3	4
Closure:	Summarized session	1	2	3	4
Overall:		1	2	3	4

What happened in the session? Concentrate on what actually took place.

What did I do which helped the students learn (before and during the session)?

What do I need to improve next time I teach?

Designing a student evaluation form

- The form should be designed based on the rules for effective feedback, i.e. as close as possible to the event, specific rather than general comments, constructive, behaviours you can change rather than personality attributes that are unchangeable (see Chapter 4).
- Outline your specific objectives for the evaluation, for example is it to check you have met your objectives (i.e. delivered what you said you would) and/or to check that the way you delivered it is acceptable?
- Consider the data entry and analysis implications of the questions you ask, and how you will use the information in your final evaluation. If in doubt, keep forms short and to the point.
- The form should begin with a brief explanation of why they are being asked to complete it and what you intend to do with the results. It should also reassure them about confidentiality and if appropriate anonymity.
- The form should include a balance of 'closed' questions such as rating scales which are easy to analyse and use for comparisons and more probing 'open' questions which seek more in-depth explanations and are generally more helpful to teacher development.
- With rating scales an odd number (e.g. 1–5 or 1–3) encourages a centring effect—some students exhibit a strong preference for the middle value. An even number on a scale (e.g. 1–4) forces student to make a more active decision. Students need some guidance as to what each value represents, and this is most simply done by labelling each extremity of the scale. For example:

	not at all valuable			very valuable
Overall the session was	1	2	3	4

- Open questions should encourage students to be specific and constructive in identifying what went well or poorly. For example:

  'What areas do you think we can improve on next time and *why*?'
- Questions should be directed at areas you can change. For example there is no point asking their opinions about space in a cramped teaching room that you can't change, but it may be worth asking given the limitations in space, is there anything they would recommend that could make it more comfortable for them?

Student evaluation form

Please help to improve your teaching by completing this form. All information will be confidential.

Teacher name ______________________ **Session title** __________________

Please rate the following	*Not at all*			*Excellent*
Overall:				
Were your learning needs met?	1	2	3	4
Was the session interesting?	1	2	3	4
Was the session useful?	1	2	3	4
Was the whole group included?	1	2	3	4
	Poor			*Excellent*
Specifically:				
The pace of the session was	1	2	3	4
The difficulty level of the session was	1	2	3	4
The teacher's use of questions was	1	2	3	4
Explanations were	1	2	3	4
The quality of visual aids was	1	2	3	4
The organization of the session was	1	2	3	4

What were good features of the teaching and why?

What did the teacher do that helped you to learn?

How could the teaching be improved?

Most teachers concentrate on the negative—remember to include enough opportunities for students to reinforce positive behaviours too. For example ask them why a particular session went well.

Your performance in teaching assessments

This happens rarely in medical education but you may come across it as an informal or formal part of teacher training courses. Most teachers are anxious about the prospect of doing this but we have found it is consistently rated one of the most useful parts to attending a training course on teaching. The type of assessments that you are likely to encounter include: formally observed 'microteaches', usually on a subject of your choice that you have prepared beforehand, structured teaching assessments with a standardized learner, assessment of teaching plans, and assessment of reflections on an observed teaching session. A sample teaching assessment form is shown overleaf. This can be used on a training course or as an aide memoire when you are observing another teacher's session.

Peer observation or review

Your peers are an excellent untapped source of feedback on your teaching. Getting a colleague you feel comfortable with to observe your teaching and give you some feedback is extremely useful. Many institutions now have formal procedures for peer review and evaluation of teaching. Ideally this is best organized in a circular fashion where each teacher gets reviewed by a colleague at the same level of experience and each teacher themselves reviews someone else in the same way. For example:

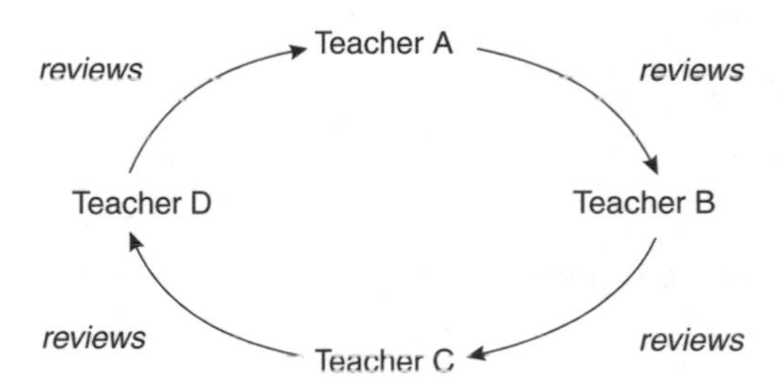

Figure 11.2 Example of a circular peer review

There is considerable value to be gained from reviewing someone else's teaching as well as having your own reviewed. The fact that it is peer-led by people who are going through the same process themselves rather than by your seniors can make the process less threatening. It is important that some basic ground rules are used to ensure that the process is constructive and 'safe' for all concerned. We have listed some ground rules for peer evaluation below. The most important of these is that the process should be led by the person who is being observed—thus if you are being observed, it should be you who sets the objectives and defines the goals in a preliminary meeting and then leads in the feedback process. It helps to use a framework for observing the session—for example the teacher assessment form overleaf.

The observer should encourage the teacher to set themselves goals for improvements for next time they teach.

Teaching assessment form

Name ________________ **Date** ____________

Session title ______________________________

Please tick if observed **Comments**

Rapport/manner

☐ Sets mood

☐ Non-verbal communication

☐ Involves patient

Student centredness

☐ Checks prior knowledge

☐ Checks past experience

☐ Checks students understanding

☐ Allows student to try and retry

☐ Involves whole group

Content

☐ Covers curriculum

☐ Knowledge base

Skills teaching

☐ Demonstrates procedure

☐ Breaks skill in parts

Micro-teaching skills

☐ Questioning skills

☐ Explaining skill

☐ Gives feedback positive/specific

☐ Uses teaching aids/variety

☐ Uses time well

Lesson structure

☐ Outlines objective

☐ Puts skill in context

☐ Plans intro/body/summary, etc.

☐ Summarizes

Reflection/self-evaluation

☐ Realistic assessment

☐ Compares well with assessors

Global assessment

Ground rules for peer evaluation

- The teacher being observed takes the lead at all times.
- Observer and teacher meet beforehand to agree ground rules (when and what to observe, how it will be undertaken, e.g. using checklist, video, confidentiality, etc.).
- Clear objectives for the observation are set beforehand.
- The process is confidential and the observer should not share his or her feelings, observations, or report with anyone else unless agreed by the teacher being observed.
- The process should not be linked to external issues such as accreditation or promotion.
- Students in the session should be briefed as to who the observer is and why they are there.
- During the session the observer will be non-participatory unless otherwise agreed by the teacher being observed.
- Feedback after the session should be as close to the event as is possible.
- The rules for effective feedback should be observed (see Chapter 4).

Mentoring and appraisal

Many teachers find it helpful to discuss their experiences with colleagues or another interested party. Co-mentoring with a colleague in a similar situation, or using a more formal appraisal system with your supervisor if you have one are two ways of doing this. These are discussed further in Chapter 12.

Course, programme, or firm evaluation

This section refers to the evaluation of courses, educational programmes, or firms. These educational activities may vary from a series of lectures to a typical clinical attachment or firm. They can include teaching a single student through to a few hundred in a lecture for a whole undergraduate year. The teaching activities may be in any setting, community or hospital and at any level, from a preclinical attachment of a few days through to training programmes for a year or more for Specialist Registrars or GP registrars.

Why do a course review?

Doing a course review is time-consuming, but it will give you valuable information about the relevance and efficiency of your course. Good courses evaluate themselves continuously, and many medical schools make sure this happens by a process of teaching governance, demanding a formal review of courses on a regular basis. To make your formal review as easy as possible it is important that the administrative side of the evaluation is well organized. Keep all course documentation and evaluation forms in order. Check with the medical school on the structure of the review required, when and to whom you should submit it (usually the curriculum committee).

It is helpful to construct your course evaluation around the headings recommended by the Teaching Quality Assessment conducted by the bodies such as the quality assurance agency (QAA) or the GMC, as this will make your next quality assurance review much easier (see box below and section on institutional evaluation following).

Areas assessed by the Quality Assurance Agency

1. Curriculum design, content, and organization.
2. Teaching, learning, and assessment.
3. Student progression and achievement.
4. Student support and guidance.
5. Learning resources.
6. Quality management and enhancement.

Techniques for a course review

A course usually involves more than one teacher, runs over a certain length of time, and is often assessed. As a result it is more complex to evaluate than the activities of a single teacher. It is important to reflect not just on the performance of each individual teacher, but on the overall course content, assessment techniques, and learning materials, and how these fit together to produce the most effective learning programme. A range of approaches is generally needed. Compiling information from all the parties involved using a range of techniques is necessary to understand not only whether a course is working but also *how* and *why* it is working. Gaining information from multiple sources using different techniques is known as 'triangulation' and is important to reduce the likelihood of knee-jerk reactions to isolated pieces of feedback. Triangulation will allow you to see if changes truly need to happen. This would be the case if all your sources of evaluation have picked up the same problem, but not if only one group of students or teachers commented on an issue that was non-recurrent. A list of some of the appropriate methods that can be employed is shown below.

Methods for course, programme, or firm evaluation

- Individual evaluations for each teacher or each session with students.
- Course evaluation form.
- Overview of curriculum, course objectives, organization, and main assessments.
- Review of individual session objectives in conjunction with course objectives.
- Reflection on the other key areas included in the Teaching Quality Assurance exercise, including ongoing course monitoring, student progression, student support, and available resources.

Individual evaluations for each teacher/session with students

Clearly individual evaluations are important, but it is also important to retain a picture of the whole course or firm. Some comparisons can be made across different teachers or sessions, but mean scores on rating scales should be interpreted cautiously as they do not give insights into why some sessions or teachers are rated particularly well or poorly. It is worth stepping back from individual teachers or sessions and seeing if any trends are apparent—for example, how do the different modes of teaching compare? Do the students prefer bedside teaching sessions on the ward or in surgery, more formal seminar teaching, or participation in teaching outpatient clinics? In the 'open' comments written by students are there any trends on aspects in the high rated sessions they found particularly helpful, or in the low rated sessions they found unhelpful?

Course evaluation form

Rather than putting together a mass of evaluation forms for each session it is certainly simpler (and more popular with students) to get them to complete one evaluation form at the end of their course or attachment with you. If you can complement this with some sort of verbal feedback from the students you will get even better quality evaluation. There are problems however with evaluating at the end of a course. The information you get on each component of the course may be of lower quality, the length of form required to cover all areas is off-putting, and evaluations may be affected by students' incomplete memory of events. Students tend to evaluate the session they have just completed higher than previous sessions where they have had a greater chance to reflect about its content and value. Also students like to see things change because of evaluation. Getting feedback at the end of the course means there is little gain for that particular group of students as the course is over.

Your registry or undergraduate office may have a standard form that students are required to complete. If you are able to design your own student evaluations it is worth thinking through the appropriate balance between evaluating individual sessions and overall course evaluation. To avoid students completing a form every time they have any educational session you could group together sessions in small clusters of four to five. Alternatively you could have a mid-point evaluation in addition to the usual end-of-course evaluation where students rate early sessions in their course or attachment and also have the opportunity to express any unmet learning needs. You will then be able to adjust the remainder of your course in the light of the information you receive.

The content of an overall course evaluation form will be different from an individual session form as it will focus less on the educational content and process of individual sessions and more on broader aspects of teaching and learning including other factors such as administration, environment, assessments, and so on. Some practical tips on designing an effective end-of-course evaluation form have been detailed below. Remember that complex forms take a long time to analyse, and you will need to clarify with your medical education unit who is to do the data entry and analysis. If you have doubts about the administration time available to you, it is wise to keep the forms reasonably succinct.

Designing an effective course evaluation form

- With the course team, consider the purpose of the form—is it purely for internal use for course development or are there also external uses (such as for the TQA)? If so, are there additional aspects that need to be included?
- Roughly outline the content in terms of broad areas you want to cover in the form—a good starting point is to look at your overall course objectives and

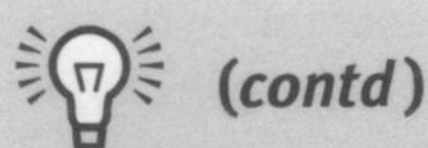

to think more broadly about the six main areas investigated by the Quality Assurance Agency. This will ensure you consider general aspects such as student support systems as well as those more directly related to your learning and teaching programme.

- Consider the data entry and analysis implications of the questions you ask, and how you will use the information in your final evaluation. If in doubt, keep forms short and to the point.
- Start the form with a brief explanation what it is and why it is important. Students should be reassured about confidentiality and if appropriate anonymity. Follow the guidance on students evaluation form design, and mix closed and open questions and rating scales. With a course evaluation form it is appropriate to see to what degree the aims and objectives of the course have been met, and open questions can identify what went well or less well and how the course can be improved.
- Consider asking more detailed questions about changes you have made to the course, or areas where you may need more resource investment.
- Rather than asking about each teaching session over the whole course you could group the sessions under broader headings such as into different types of teaching, e.g. lectures, seminars, small group teaching, or different settings, e.g. clinics, bedside teaching, operating theatre, domiciliary visits, or different teachers within the course/firm. Alternatively you could simply ask them to name the best and worst sessions in the course with the reasons why they have selected these particular ones.

Course meeting

Once some of the basic data has been gathered from the students you will need to collect data from the teachers. If the course is large or covers multiple sites you may have to do this using a form, but if possible it is helpful to have a minuted meeting of all the course teachers to discuss the course covering the following areas:

Overview of curriculum, course objectives, and main assessments. This is about the bigger picture and making sure all components fit together.

- Has your course achieved its stated objectives?
- Are all important areas of the curriculum contained within the course?
- Does your main assessment test your main objectives? For example, if you use problem orientated or problem-based learning as your main teaching method, does your assessment test their problem solving skills as well as factual recall?
- How have the students performed on the assessments?
- Were there any particular areas where they performed less well and have they failed to meet any of the objectives?

Review of individual session objectives in conjunction with course objectives. This involves checking on how the different teaching encounters relate to each other and making sure they complete the whole picture. Are general course objectives being addressed in the individual session objectives? Is there any unhelpful repetition? Are there any gaps? The 'generic' skills objectives such as history taking or communication skills are commonly omitted in reviews of overall objectives. A useful way of ensuring your curriculum contains all major topics as well as generic competencies is to construct a blueprint (as discussed in Chapter 9, p. 152) to use as a checklist with your topics as rows and competencies as columns. A sample grid showing a small part of a psychiatry course is shown below.

	Knowledge	Application knowledge/ problem solving	History taking	Mental state exam	Communication skills
Psychosis and mania					
Depression and suicide					
Anxiety, panic disorder somatization, and phobias					
The older patient: acute/ chronic confusion					

If you designed the course you probably started off with a grid like this to ensure that the students were going to cover all the aims and objectives you had planned. Use the blueprint to plot the content of each session as it actually took place, and check that what you planned actually matched what was taught.

Consideration of broader support of learning. Moving away from the learning and teaching encounters themselves, it is important to consider other equally important but more frequently neglected areas, such as available resources, student support systems, quality assurance processes, and staff development. This is an area that is often neglected at course level, as many teachers feel it forms part of a departmental or institutional evaluation. If there are issues that materially affect your course, it is wise to include them in your report.

Writing a course report

The course report is the summary of all your evaluation efforts. Your medical school may request a particular format, and it is wise to check with colleagues the detail and length that is expected of you. Include a description of the course as it was planned, and as it was delivered, with explanations for the divergence between the two. Include estimates of staff time and resource use to enable the school to estimate cost, and student assessments and evaluations to show how effective you have been.

Putting together the findings of an evaluation is time-consuming. Make sure that you have enough time to complete your work, and that once it is done you circulate the results as widely as possible.

Departmental and institutional evaluation

Just as a course or firm is more than the activity of one teacher, so the activities of a department and institution are more then the sum of the individual courses. Any evaluation has to take into account the interaction between the courses, the faculty, and the available resources. In order to make institutions more easily comparable, the government recently introduced the Teaching Quality Assessment (TQA) exercise conducted by the Quality Assurance Agency (QAA). This is a bit like an OFSTED inspection of a school but for higher education institutions. This looks at the activities of an institution under a series of headings (see box below). The TQA is important for several reasons. First, poor results lead to remediation, which is stressful for the institution, the teachers, and the students. Secondly, the results are freely available, and prospective students can gauge the position of one course against another and decide whether they would like to attend an institution or not. Prospective teaching staff can also use the results to decide whether they would like to work in the institution or not. However, as yet the TQA does not have the ability to reward highly performing institutions in the way that the Research Assessment Exercise (RAE) does.

Teaching Quality Assessment (TQA) headings

Curriculum design, content, and organization. This looks at the content and structure of the curriculum. It compares the written curriculum to the 'real' curriculum experienced by students, and the organizational support provided for teachers.

Teaching, learning, and assessment. This examines the quality of teaching and learning materials. Assessment procedures are examined for reliability and validity.

Student progression and achievement. This assesses students progression both within and after the course.

Student support and guidance. This deals with the institutions capacity to support student learning and any pastoral problems which may arise.

Learning resources. This assesses the adequacy of buildings, libraries, and equipment.

Quality management and enhancement. This deals with the institutions ability to monitor the quality of its courses and to develop the teaching skills of staff.

Performing a departmental or institution evaluation is very complex, and beyond the scope of this book (see Further reading).

If you have already taken part in a quality assurance exercise, you will know that it entails a lot of work for every teaching department in a medical school. Your evaluations of your course will be a part of the final submission, but you may have to rework your reports. To keep this work to a minimum it is worth trying to stay up-to-date, keeping electronic copies of your data and reports, and filing all information carefully. As mentioned previously, structuring your final evaluations of your course following the headings laid out by the TQA will make integration of your work into the final submission easier.

What to do with a poor evaluation

The first point to remember is that it happens to the best of us—we can't be everything for everyone all of the time. It is important though to reflect on why your poor evaluation has occurred on this particular occasion. There are likely to be a number of interacting factors, some of which may be out of your control.

External factors affecting teaching

Common factors affecting evaluations that frequently appear beyond the control of the individual teacher include:

The topic. Some topics are unpopular with students, and it is hard to motivate them. Topics which are perceived to have low relevance and utility do not engage students and they are likely to rate the session poorly. Students will be more highly motivated by topics that have immediate relevance to them (and their exams—see below) and if this does not apply to your topic then it is worthwhile putting extra thought into how you can help students see the relevance of what they are doing. Students rate sessions poorly that are not at the right pitch for them. It may be the nature of the topic you have been asked to teach is pitched either too high or too low for the students, and you could liaise with other course tutors, the overall course, or curriculum leader to adapt this.

Assessment does not relate to the learning methods. As described in Chapter 9, assessment is one of the strongest driving forces for motivating learning, particularly for undergraduates. If students perceive that what they are learning, or the way in which they are learning it is not relevant for their exam then their motivation, learning, and your evaluation will be affected. If you find yourself in this position, the first step would be to approach the person involved in setting the students assessments. You should discuss how the examination or other assessments could be adapted to integrate your topic. You could also consider how you might integrate formative assessments into your own teaching session. There are few things that motivate an audience to pay attention more than saying 'I'm going to give you a quiz on this at the end'.

Environmental factors. Common problems in all medical schools include overcrowding, poorly heated/ventilated or inappropriate rooms, or having a teaching slot at the end of a long morning before everyone has lunch. If these can be anticipated then it is worth considering what can be done to improve things, or at the least show that you care about student welfare. For example, asking for extra heaters or fans to be supplied, providing refreshments, or allowing time in your planning for a quick coffee/toilet break will revive flagging students and improve your evaluation.

Last minute teaching. Having to take on teaching for a colleague at the last minute is a common scenario, and using someone else's acetates/slides/lesson plan is rarely as effective as using your own. Another common scenario where lack of time is a key factor is in opportunistic teaching settings, where you are expected to teach around a busy clinical workload. Ways you can improve on teaching in such settings have been specifically addressed in Chapter 8 on Teaching in the service setting.

Student factors. The individual or group you are teaching may be particularly uninterested in your topic, or may have personal concerns affecting their motivation and hence evaluation of your session. It is good practice to try and address these issues during the session by reading students verbal and non-verbal cues. If students appear bored/restless/disinterested/asleep during a session then it is worth stopping briefly to confront the problem. This will also give you opportunity to vary the stimulus (see Chapters 3 and 4). For example you might say 'You seem a bit restless, lets take a short two minute break. In this time can you think about what parts of this topic you would particularly like to address in the remainder of the session'. If appropriate, particularly in one to one settings, you may also want to address personal concerns that are affecting a students attention and motivation.

Teacher factors affecting teaching

Other factors leading to a poor evaluation relate more to the individual teacher. Examples of this include:

Your mood. We all have our 'off days', and personal concerns can easily erode into professional lives. Acknowledgement of your situation to yourself and others often helps relieve some of the additional distress and consequences.

Poor preparation. The importance of preparation has already been addressed in Chapter 3. Very few people can get away with 'winging it' on the day and taking time to prepare adequately for teaching is always rewarded.

Performance anxiety. Many people are anxious 'performing' in front of students, particularly larger audiences. First, it is important not to be too self-critical and to separate the 'performance' from the 'person'—i.e. a poor performance is no reflection on you as a person. A key step to reducing performance anxiety is practise—to yourself at home in front of a mirror, to your family or friends, your colleagues—anyone willing to listen. Feeling confident with the content of your lesson plan helps with the delivery on the day. There are other techniques that can be used such as 'visualization' where you imagine yourself in the situation beforehand. If performance anxiety is a real concern of yours consider attending a presentation skills course.

Presentation skills. This includes aspects such as projection and modulation of your voice, reducing performance anxiety, setting the right pace, effective use of audio-visual aids. Most major academic institutions run courses on presentation skills and there are many commercially available courses run for business people that are easily transferable to the educational setting.

Interaction. Attention span is limited where there is no change in stimulation and promoting interaction is a key way of stimulating interest and promoting learning. This has been addressed in further detail in Chapter 4.

Pitch. A common complaint from students is that the session is pitched either too high for them and not relevant to their needs, or too low and seems slow, repetitive, and even patronizing. The best way to avoid either scenario is to make an effort to get to know your audience—what stage are they at in their attachment, what teaching have they had on this topic before, what do they want to know about this area? You will not always have this information in advance—if not, then ask the students at the start of the session and be prepared to be flexible and change your pitch according to their needs.

Poor motivation. This may be that you are not motivated yourself to teach on this topic—in which case consider asking a colleague to swap or rotate with you. Alternatively it may be that students have not been sufficiently motivated to learn, a key component of the introduction of the session we have discussed further in Chapter 3.

You may be able to identify problem(s) yourself by reflecting on and correcting causes as listed above. If you are not clear about the problem, it is worth asking a supportive colleague to sit in on your session and feedback on your teaching skills. Once you have identified a problem, you may be able to remedy it yourself by changing your objectives, teaching method, or time allocation during the session. However, it is often helpful to seek outside support. This may be by attending courses to brush up on your teaching skills, peer support or mentoring, through staff appraisal schemes, or contacting your institution's staff development officer. These will be discussed further in Chapter 12.

Summary

Evaluation is a key activity for all teachers. On a personal level it can help to improve your teaching, and help you develop as a teacher. To get an accurate result, information needs to be collected from as many sources as possible, and it needs to be sufficiently detailed for teachers to understand how to improve teaching.

Evaluating courses uses the same principles as evaluating individual teaching sessions, although information is collected from a wider range of sources and includes data from administrative as well as academic sources. With the introduction of the TQA, the evaluation of teaching has become very important for institutions. Structuring all your evaluation activities with the needs of the external evaluation in mind is wise.

References

Dent, J. A., and Harden, R. (2001) *A practical guide for medical teachers*. Edinburgh: Churchill Livingstone.

Kirkpatrick, D. I. (1967) Evaluation of training. In *Training and development handbook* (ed. R. Craig and I. Bittel). New York: McGraw-Hill.

Newble, D., and Cannon, R. (1994) *A handbook for medical teachers*, 3rd edn. London: Kluwer Academic Publishers.

Ramsden, R. (1992) *Learning to teach in higher education*. London: Routledge.

Rippey, R. M. (1981) *The evaluation of teaching in medical schools*. New York: Springer Publishing Company.

Snell, L., Tallett, S., Haist, S., Hays, R., Norcini, J., Prince, K., *et al.* (2000) A review of the evaluation of clinical teaching: new perspectives and challenges. *Med Educ* **34**, 862–70.

Wilkes, M., and Bligh, J. (1999) Evaluating educational interventions. *Br Med J* **318**, 1269–72.

Further reading

Rippey, R. M. (1981) *The evaluation of teaching in medical schools*. New York: Springer Publishing Company.

The Quality Assurance Agency. *A handbook for academic review*. Linney Direct, Adamsway, Mansfield, Nottinghamshire: QAA (downloadable from www.qaa.ac.uk)

CHAPTER 12
Developing as a teacher

'*While we teach we learn*' Seneca Epistolae VII. viii.

To have read this far in the book you will already be a motivated and dedicated teacher, who is keen to deliver a good quality product. Hopefully this book will have equipped you with some of the tools to teach more effectively and efficiently. In this chapter we will explore things a little more and look at the possible pathways and opportunities to develop your skills further.

Why develop as a teacher?

Teaching is a responsibility few of us take lightly. We are training '*Tomorrow's Doctors*'. In the current climate of accountability and professional development, those who teach have a responsibility to develop and maintain their teaching skills. Professionalization encompasses the professional training, behaviours, and attitudes that promote high quality education.

No one would expect a teacher in any other environment to begin teaching without any training or supervision but that is what often happens in medical education. Medical teachers are often employed by trusts rather than medical schools and they can often see little in the way of reward for providing high quality teaching. Pathways for those keen to teach can seem somewhat unclear. Academic departments still seem to prize research before teaching and so becoming an academic may not always be the answer. However, if you are fitting teaching into a clinical role, even in a teaching hospital or practice, it can often be relegated to second place behind clinical commitments. So how can we ensure learning and teaching gets the recognition and rewards it deserves?

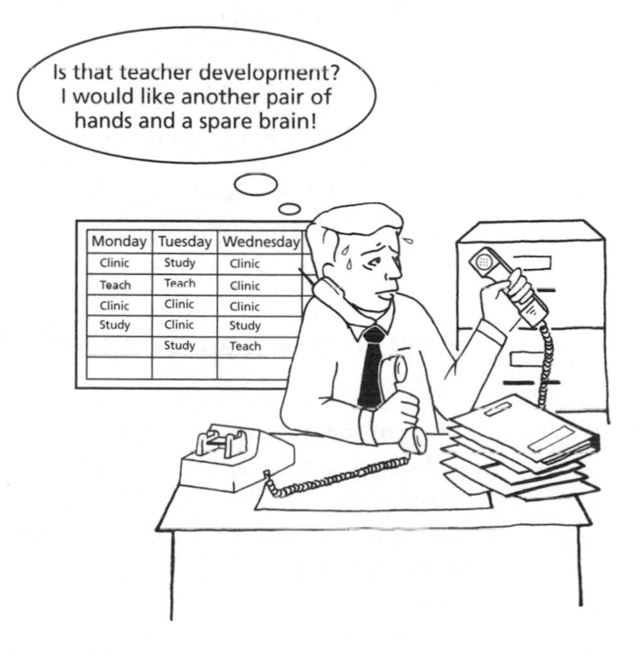

Changes in the socio-political and professional climate are beginning to favour the medical teacher. General Medical Council recommendations in *Duties of a doctor* (GMC, 1998) and *The doctor as teacher* (GMC, 1999) have now outlined very clearly what is expected of all doctors with regard to teaching. The new consultant contract and revalidation processes emphasize lifelong professional development and accountability. These changes affect all of those who teach, whether they are employed teaching staff or those who fit teaching into a clinical workload.

Quality assurance in the wider field of higher education has also begun to have more teeth in recent years and this trend is now influencing those who provide medical education.

The Dearing Report into higher education (Dearing, 1997) has had widespread effects on the provision of good quality teaching and the recognition and reward for those who deliver this teaching. The report has spawned an important development that will have a very significant influence on medical teachers and their institutions: the Quality Assurance Agency. The effect the quality assurance agency will have on medical education will be mainly at an institutional level. The knock-on effects on individual teachers will be twofold: at last some recognition of good educational practices, but also an increased scrutiny and accountability. It is in the interest of all medical teachers to ensure they make the most of the opportunities that allow them to develop and flourish in this environment.

Why develop as a teacher?

Personal

For a sense of personal satisfaction.

For reaccredidation purposes.

Retention and promotion.

Being able to do things well often removes much of the stress.

For the student

Better teachers help make learning happen.

Better face to face teaching and better programmes, courses, and assessments.

Better value for money.

For the institution

For quality assurance purposes.

A reputation as a centre of teaching excellence—to attract students and high quality staff.

How to develop as a medical teacher

There are a variety of ways to develop as a medical teacher. If you have just read some of the proceeding chapters that is one of them! You can also develop your skills at a personal level by practising the skills of being a reflective teacher and by maintaining a teaching portfolio. These will help you to think about how you teach and how you could improve. You can also get help from others: either your peers or from formal staff development opportunities. Some teachers choose to take up academic or teaching post or study for higher qualifications in teaching. All of these activities encourage us to keep up-to-date, to reflect, and to engage in continuing professional development. In this way we are *professionalizing* what we do. This can only be a good thing, both for your own personal sense of achievement but also for the institutions and ultimately the students we serve.

The reflective practitioner

In the previous chapter we looked at how to evaluate your teaching by developing the skills of reflection on the teaching process. This can be done formally or informally. The benefits of doing this formally is that you have documented what went well, what worked, what didn't work, and you can plan changes for the next time you teach. You can compare your performance in subsequent sessions to see how you have improved. You will also have evidence that you have spent some time reflecting on your performance. This sort of evidence is used in Quality Assurance procedures and will be useful in a reaccredidation portfolio.

You could devise your own checklist based around what you hope to achieve, and then review it after a set period of time. This helps you to focus on what is important to you, and will give you a sense of achievement. Some aims you won't have achieved and it is tempting just to roll them to the next checklist. However, it is worth considering why you did not achieve them—your circumstances may have changed, training opportunities were not available, or you didn't have enough time. When you write your next checklist you might want to include them, amend them, or omit them altogether.

Producing and maintaining a teaching portfolio

Most teachers are unclear about what a teaching portfolio actually is and how it is used. Teaching portfolios have recently come into vogue in medical education and should be thought of like an artist's portfolio. An artist includes in his portfolio examples of his best work, work that reflects the range of his abilities, and which he is happy to show to others.

A teaching portfolio usually includes two elements: a reflective document on *how* you teach and *why*, plus evidence to support your claims.

Producing a reflective document may seem a little alien to the medical teacher. This is not something that we have been asked to do before. It encourages you to reflect on all the teaching and support of learning activities you are involved with to try and identify the strategy for the methods and approaches you adopt. Hopefully these strategies will fit in with recent trends in medical education or be based on evidence. If they do not, outline the reasons why not and the ways in which you feel things could improve. The document should be about everything you do with regard education; undergraduate and postgraduate, face to face teaching, and the other activities that support teaching such as curriculum activity work, course evaluation meetings, promoting an effective learning environment.

The gathering of evidence section may seem like a cumbersome and tedious task but an up-to-date portfolio is becoming increasingly important in appointments, promotion, quality assurance visits, and revalidation. Collecting the evidence as you go along reduces the stress of trying to gather evidence for interviews, appraisals, etc.

Many of the sections in this chapter discuss producing reflective documents and evidence of good teaching. There is an enormous degree of overlap. You will find that keeping one relatively comprehensive set of evidence and producing and updating one reflective document will serve almost every purpose.

> Start a box file today. Label it 'Teaching Portfolio' and start gathering evidence regularly. Include student evaluations, notes from observers of your teaching, thank you letters from learners and course organizers, etc. It will form the 'supporting evidence' for your portfolio and will take the pressure off trying to find dozens of documents at short notice.

Appraisal and professional development plans

Within medical education the boundaries between educational supervisors, appraisers, evaluators, and mentors are often blurred with the same person frequently adopting more than one role. Your supervisor should have most of the attributes shown in the box below to be able to help you.

The idea behind appraisal is for you and your supervisor to put aside some time to reflect on your achievements and to shape your planned professional development over a time period, usually of a year or two. Most medical teachers are familiar with appraisal of their development as health professionals, but our development as teachers is frequently overlooked. This means you are missing out on recognition of a significant part of your work and also that any training and development opportunities for you as a teacher are missed. A way to be systematic about an appraisal covering all areas of your work is to keep a professional development plan. This lays out how you want to develop over a forthcoming period of time and how you might achieve those goals. Always include your development goals as a teacher. The framework of a professional development plan over a number of years is also useful when constructing other reflective documents or providing evidence of achievement.

Attributes of a doctor with responsibilities for clinical training/education supervision (General Medical Council, 1999)

An enthusiasm for his/her speciality.

A personal commitment to teaching and learning.

Sensitivity and responsiveness to the educational needs of junior doctors.

Capacity to promote development of the required professional attitudes and values.

An understanding of the principles of education as applied to medicine.

An understanding of research methods.

Practical teaching skills.

A willingness to develop as both a doctor and a teacher.

A commitment to audit and peer review of his/her teaching.

The ability to use formative assessment for the benefit of the trainee.

The ability to carry out formal appraisal of the performance of the trainee as a practicing doctor.

Mentoring

The Homeric concept of the mentor is that of a wise counsellor, a good friend, and a role model. The term mentor has traditionally been used in the business sector to describe powerful individuals who take a protégé under their wings with the aim of using their power and influence to shape and advance that persons career. When we use it in the educational setting, we imply something to do with the provision of support and being a suitable role model. Within the field of medical education, the standing Committee on Postgraduate Medical and Dental Education have described a mentor as one who:

> '. . . . *guides another individual (the mentee) in the development and re-examination of their own ideas, learning, and personal and professional development.*'
>
> (SCOPME, 1998)

The key activities of a mentor can be described as providing academic, personal, and professional support to the mentee. As you can see there may be some difficulty if the same person is providing the mentoring support, is running your appraisals, and is in charge of hiring and firing you!

Having a mentoring relationship is enormously fulfilling and helps you to make wise and appropriate decisions about your teaching career.

Choosing a mentor is a highly personal thing but a number of issues need to be considered whomever you ask to be your mentor. First, mentoring is time-consuming, and your potential mentor will need the time and commitment to the role. To reduce the time commitment it is easier if you are geographically close. Secondly, they will need to understand and respect both the purpose and process of mentoring. Thirdly, they must understand the nature and breadth of your teaching, and finally they will need to be a friend, someone with whom one can share failures as well as successes. It is sensible to reach agreement at an early stage about issues around the boundaries of the relationship. Both of you will need to constantly reflect on the remit of the relationship and consider situations when another person or role is more suitable to deal with an issue.

Mentoring has become popular over the last decade despite a lack of evidence for its value in the medical educational literature. It is seen as a solution to some of the education and support problems posed by the changes in service provision (SCOPME, 1998). The literature is currently at the exploratory and descriptive stages (Jowers and Herr, 1990), although there are some positive evaluations (Alliot, 1996; Illes *et al.*, 2000; Morzinski *et al.*, 1996). The rationale for mentoring is drawn from its potential enhancement of the reflective element in experiential learning (Kolb, 1984; Schön, 1987). The process of mentoring has been described, and four phases of the mentoring relationship are recognized: initiation (establishing rapport), setting direction, development, and finalizing/maintenance (Megginson and Clutterbuck, 1995). While mentors are generally more senior than their mentee there is no rigid criteria for their selection. The key feature is that mentor and mentee can establish a working relationship. However the mentor needs confidence (in giving clear directions, allowing the mentee to take the initiative, and in the limitations of their knowledge), commitment (to training and developing their mentee), and competence (in their field, and in communication skills) (Morton-Cooper and Palmer, 2002). Training for mentors and ongoing support for mentors is desirable (Ferguson, 1995), and the status of mentoring raised by linking it to the nominations and appointments process.

Peer observation and support

Your peers can be an important untapped source of support in your aim towards improving as a teacher. The most important thing about using peer observation and support is to ensure that the individuals *are* actually peers. They don't have to do the same clinical job as you but they should be at the same stage of development as a teacher. Peer relationships can be utilized either as observers of each others teaching sessions or as a sounding board for your ideas and exasperation.

Peer observation

Many institutions now encourage peer observation in the teaching process. The easiest way to arrange it is to find a time when the observer can sit in on some of your teaching. This needs to be supplemented with a meeting some time before the session both to highlight the areas you would most like feedback on and to establish the ground rules. The observed session also needs to be followed up as soon as possible with a chance for the observer to feedback on the session. Where possible this verbal feedback should be supported with some written comments. This set-up is simple and can be reciprocated at a later date with the observer doing the teaching. However in this arrangement the parties often know each other very well and there is a tendency for things to get a little cosy or for observers not being critical enough in order to spare the others feelings. A way around this is to use a peer observation snake whereby teacher A observes teacher B who observes teacher C and so on.

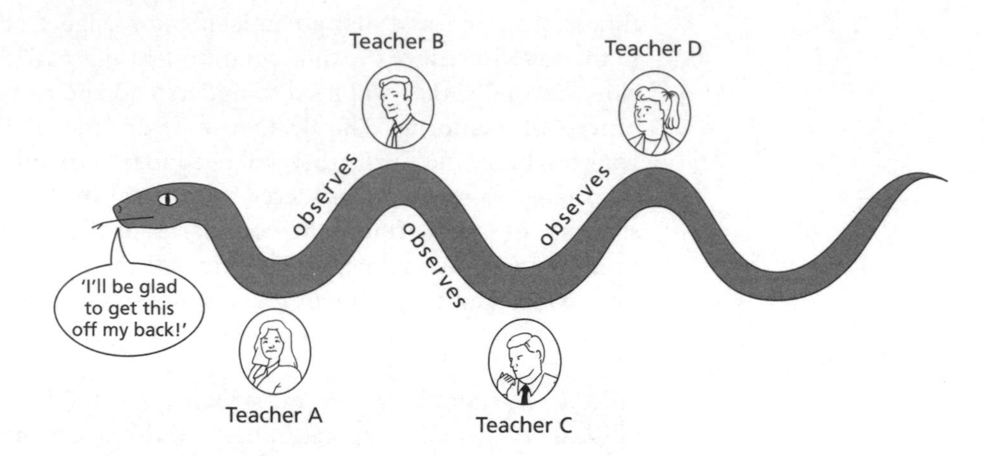

In this way you can get a large number of teachers involved and can place yourself in the snake next to someone you know less well. Peer observation, like any feedback activity, needs some ground rules to ensure maximum benefit.

Suggested peer observation ground rules

Make it a confidential process.

Plan ahead:
Allow time for briefing.
Choose a suitable session.
Clarify any particular areas to focus on.

Make sure the teacher and students know what is happening.

Introduce the observer to the students and clarify their role.

Arrange time for feedback as soon as possible after the session.

Use the rules of constructive feedback to discuss the session.

Peer support

Teachers can offer each other support in other ways apart from directly observing the teaching process. At a very informal level, peer support can mean a couple of teachers looking at each others lesson plans, sharing experiences of good and bad teaching sessions, and sharing resources. Setting aside a time and place to meet with a larger number of peers can be a useful way of exploring ideas, sharing good practice, critical incident analysis, sharing information about staff development courses, or just having a chat about where people are at. Think of it as what might happen in the staffroom with schoolteachers. These meetings can be informal or formal. The advantage of making them formal is that they can be minuted and actions suggested.

This can go into your teaching portfolio as evidence of reflection but more importantly it can inform those at strategic levels about the experiences and suggestions of the teachers at the chalk face. Having the support of your peers cannot be underestimated in situations such as medical teaching where teaching activity is sporadic, fragmented, and often unsupported.

Staff development and teaching courses

Your institution probably provides formal training courses to support the development of professional skills including teaching skills. Past models of staff development for health professionals have either focused on an 'on-the-job learning'/'baptism of fire' approach or consisted of uncoordinated, ill-conceived short courses. This has done little to encourage the teacher to develop his or her skills. With our increased accountability, more effective staff development activities have been developed and in many cases your staff development department will help you realize your development plans.

Staff development courses may be an opportunity to meet colleagues from other fields or institutions and are a good way to develop links with peers. They often take place in protected time away from service delivery in order to focus and reflect on the teaching process. Almost every institution or organization will have a staff development and training unit that can advise you of courses aimed at teaching skills. Alternatively courses may be advertised in the mainstream medical press.

Many medical teachers may feel that such courses are aimed at novices and indeed many courses are. However an increasing number of courses are aimed at the practicing medical teacher and are suitable for teachers from all areas of the health professions with a range of experience. A particularly common format is the 'TIPS' course (TIPS, 1976) which is usually a two day experiential workshop which focuses on equipping teachers with the tools to become effective teachers. If you are lucky enough to be linked to a university, there will be a whole range of teacher training opportunities including probationers' courses for new teachers, specialist courses such as large group teaching skills, facilitation skills, supervising project work, etc.

Finding out about the course is important before giving up your time (and sometimes money) to attend. Talk to the course organizer, and perhaps someone who has successfully completed the course.

Staff development courses are only part of a continuum that focuses on the development of the teacher as a professional. Courses are at their least useful when they take place in a vacuum. If you build staff development courses into your professional development plan and aim to attend the courses you *need* to attend as well as those you *want* to attend then you can maximize, and justify, the usefulness of courses that you attend. Offering to share your learning from these courses with your fellow department members also helps to justify your absence from the service delivery.

Further qualifications in teaching

There are a number of ways to formally recognizing your achievements in developing as a teacher. These include membership of organizations such as the Institute for Learning and Teaching in Higher Education (ILTHE), participating in courses that are accredited by one of the teaching bodies, or by taking formal teaching qualifications.

Membership of an accreditation body

The Institute for Learning and Teaching in Higher Education (ILTHE) is a membership organization that promotes good teaching practice. It was set up in the wake of the Dearing Report into higher education and it welcomes teachers from all areas of higher education. Membership is gained by a number of routes such as completing the individual application for membership process or by successfully completing an accredited course. The mission statement of the ILTHE is:

- To enhance the status of teaching in higher education.
- To maintain and improve the quality of learning and teaching in higher education.
- To set standards of good professional practice that its members, and in due course all those with learning and teaching responsibilities, might follow.

From the mission statement and admission procedures two things are clear. First, that membership of this organization should mark a teacher out as being a high quality educator committed to improving learning and teaching. Secondly, the last point in the mission statement suggests that eventually this organization, or a very similar one, will be responsible for defining the criteria for those who are involved in teaching. It is probable in the not too distant future that all higher education teachers will be expected to become members of such an organization.

For the medical teacher the benefits of membership include this tangible acknowledgement of excellence plus the opportunity to be a pioneer in shaping developments in medical education.

The Staff Development and Education Association (SEDA) is co-operative network of interested professionals and also has a fellowship scheme that offers professional accreditation for higher education teachers.

Accredited courses

We often attend courses in teaching with just CME or PGEA approval. However the wise medical teacher may look out for courses that both fulfil a learning need and that lead to some sort of accreditation. The two main accreditation bodies in the UK are the ILTHE and SEDA. Both of these organizations support and accredit a range of courses that either have credit in their own right or allow you to take up membership of the organization or gain credits towards a higher qualification.

Often such courses are longer and more detailed than staff development courses you are used to and will have some form of assessment. They may give more cohesion to your development as a teacher and should be included in your CV and teaching portfolio.

Higher qualifications in teaching

Many medical teachers now pursue higher qualifications in medical education either for a personal sense of achievement or as part of a promotion process.

Most medical education higher degrees are modular, with both a Certificate and Diploma stage proceeding the acquisition of a masters degree. The degree may be a Master of Arts (MA), a Master of Education (M Ed), or a Master of Medical Education (M MEd). The modular nature of courses means that you can opt in or out of courses as your circumstances and needs change. There are now a large number of institutions offering medical education degrees. The best known are those at the Institute of Education at the University of London which offers a taught degree course in Higher and professional education, Cardiff and Nottingham which offer a combination of taught sessions at the campus together with some independent work, and Dundee which offers a highly flexible distance learning M MEd.

All of these courses can be fitted alongside ongoing service commitment but you will need to think carefully about the time and resources such study will take up. Try to get the support of your supervisor and institution. This may help with finances, protected time to study, and with the will to continue.

For those who wish to develop their medical education expertise beyond the masters level there are a number of centres that offer both traditional PhDs in education and the educational doctorate (Ed D) which is more experiential than a traditional doctorate programme and aimed at practicing professionals.

Developing a teaching career

In this age of portfolio careers it is possible to develop your interest in teaching into a career or part of a career. Often these teaching strands to a medical career happen by being in the right place at the right time and making sure those in senior positions know about your abilities. The advertisement sections of the mainstream medical journals are a useful guide to the jobs on offer, as are the specialist medical education publications. Academic jobs with an emphasis on teaching are few and far between but are on the increase so keep your teaching portfolio up-to-date. They are often part-time and so will allow you to continue with your clinical pursuits. Membership of the ILTHE or SEDA and obtaining a higher qualification in teaching will help to make you a suitable candidate for a teaching job.

Keeping up-to-date and educational research

Part of developing in any profession involves keeping up-to-date with developments in your field. Whatever your level of involvement in teaching, reading the medical education publications is a worthwhile pursuit. It will keep you up-to-date, it will provide you with examples of good practice that you can develop in your own setting, and it will encourage you to practice evidence-based education. For a few it will inspire you to develop an educational research project. Medical education research is a relatively new field and a whole host of methodologies are used to answer research questions. It is important that as a profession we explore and evaluate new and existing ideas to develop a culture of evidence-based practice.

Many of the membership organizations produce peer-reviewed journals and arrange national and international conferences. In the UK the Association for the Study of Medical Education (ASME) produces '*Medical Education*'. The Association for Medical Education in Europe (AMEE) produces '*Medical Teacher*'. Both of these journals provide clear, well-written articles and research pieces that are interesting and will inform your practice.

Summary

There are many reasons to develop as a medical teacher, some more tangible than others. There are a range of pathways and opportunities for our activities to become more professional. The culture of medical education is rapidly changing and it is up to *us* to make the most of these changes. We need to constantly reflect on our roles as teachers and also to consider our professional development as being that of clinician *and* teacher.

References

Alliot, R. (1996) Facilitating mentoring in general practice. *Br Med J* **28**, 2–3.

Dearing, R. (1997) *Report of the national committee of enquiry into higher education.* London: HMSO.

Ferguson, L. M. (1995) Faculty support for nurse preceptors. *Nurs Connect* **8**, 37–49.

General Medical Council. (1998) *Good medical practice.* London: General Medical Practice.

General Medical Council. (1999) *The doctor as teacher.* London: General Medical Council.

Illes, J., Glover, G. H., Wexler, L., Leung, A. N., and Glazer, G. M. (2000) A model for faculty mentoring in academic radiology. *Acad Radiol* **7**, 717–24.

Jowers, L. T., and Herr, K. (1990) A review of literature on mentor-protegee relationships. *NLN Publ* 49–77.

Kolb, D. A. (1984) *Experiential learning—experience as the source of learning and development.* NJ: Englewood Cliffs.

Megginson, D., and Clutterbuck, D. (1995) *Mentoring in action.* London: Kogan Page.

Morton-Cooper, A. and Palmer, A. (2002) *Mentoring and preceptorship.* Oxford: Blackwell Science.

Morzinski, J. A., Diehr, S., Bower, D. J., and Simpson, D. E. (1996) A descriptive, cross-sectional study of formal mentoring for faculty. *Fam Med* **28**, 434–8.

Schön, D. A. (1987) *The reflective practitioner.* San Francisco: Jossey-Bass.

SCOPME (1998) *An enquiry into mentoring: supporting doctors and dentists at work.* London: Standing Committee on Medical and Dental Education.

TIPS (1976) *Teaching improvement project system.* Kentucky: The Kellogg Foundation.

Resources

The Institute of Learning and Teaching in Higher Education, Genesis 3, Innovation Way, York Science Park, Heslington, York Y010 5DQ, UK

http://www.ilt.ac.uk

SEDA, Gala House, 3 Raglan Road, Edgbaston, Birmingham B5 7RA, UK

The Association for the study of Medical Education (ASME), 12 Queen Street, Edinburgh EH2 1JE, UK

Tel: 0131 225 9111; Fax: 0131 225 9444; email: info@asme.org.uk

Web address: http://www.asme.org.uk

The Association for Medical Education in Europe (AMEE), The University of Dundee, Tay Park House, 484 Perth Road, Dundee DD2 1LR, UK

Web address: http://www.amee.org

Centre for Medical Education (Further qualifications in Medical education), The University of Dundee, Tay Park House, 484 Perth Road, Dundee DD2 1LR, UK

email: dundee.ac.uk

Institute of Education, Bedford Square, London WC1, UK

Web address: http://www.ioe.ac.uk

Cardiff, School of Medical and Dental Education, UWCM, Heath Park, Cardiff CF14 4XN, UK

Web address: http://www.uwcm.ac.uk/studt/postgraduate/index.htm

Nottingham (MMedSci in Clinical Education), Nottingham University Medical School, Room B76C Queen's Medical Centre, Nottingham NG7 2UH, UK

Tel: (0115) 970 9374; Fax: (0115) 970 9922;

email: Malcolm.pendlebury@nottingham.ac.uk

Glossary of terms and abbreviations

Active learning	Motivating and involving students with their learning.
Adult learning (Andragogy)	A range of theories initially developed by Knowles proposing that adults learn differently from children.
Advance organizer	A stimulus which is designed to cue the learners prior knowledge to enable further learning (developed by Ausubel).
Aim	A broad statement of the intent of a teaching programme.
Appraisal	A formal and regular review of work which usually encourages the learner to reflect upon their progress.
Assessment	Measuring how much students have learned.
Blueprint	A method for ensuring that the content of a course or assessment accurately reflects the original objectives.
Buzz group	Teaching technique involving splitting a large group into smaller groups for an activity.
CAL (computer-assisted learning)	Use of computers for learning.
Checklist	A technique allowing an assessor to note whether a student performed an action or not.
Clinical vignette	A short written description of a case, often used as the problem in PBL, or as a stem MCQs and EMQs.
Cognitive theory	A group of learning theories stressing the importance of the learner's interaction with information.
Competency	An action that a student is expected to perform to a certain level.
Concept mapping	A method of visually representing the different concepts and principles needed to understand a subject.
Constructivism	A theory proposing that new information is built onto old knowledge and transformed by the learner in an active process.
Course	A series of teaching sessions linked to one topic.

Criterion referencing	The use of a pre-set standard against which to assess student performance.
CRQ	Constructed response question: questions that permit free text answers (and are consequently less objective).
Curriculum	The content, teaching strategies, and delivery of the teaching programme.
Deep learning	A learning approach in which students seek to understand the information they are presented with.
Dissertation	A written report based on personal research, either original work or a literature review.
Distractor	In an MCQ or EMQ, the alternative (incorrect) answers.
Domain of learning	A particular area of learning—divided by Bloom into cognitive (knowledge), psychomotor (skills), and affective (attitudes).
Double-marking	The use of more than one examiner to assess a student, increasing objectivity.
Educational climate	Physical and psychological environment in which learning occurs.
EMQ	Extended Matching Questions: an objective method of testing knowledge objectives that allows testing of clinical reasoning.
Evaluation	Measuring the quality of teaching at session, course, or institutional level.
Evidence-based medical education	A move to increase the quality of research underpinning education, with the aim of increasing the effectiveness of teaching.
Experiential learning	Learning from experience, represented by the experiential learning cycle developed by Kolb.
Facilitation	Encouraging students to learn independently.
Feasibility	The ease with which a test can be performed.
Feedback	Advice on improving performance: constructive feedback is positive, specific, and offers suggestions for performance improvement.
Formative assessment	Assessing learning with the aim of feeding back information to the student to help them learn.
Generic competencies	Transferable skills such as team-working or communication essential to a practicing clinician.
Humanist theory	A group of learning theories developed by Maslow and Rogers, stressing the importance of motivation and personal growth of the learner.
ILT	Institute of Teaching and Learning (an organization promoting the professional development of teachers).
Independent learning	A type of learning in which the students decides the content and process of the learning and studies alone. Other terms are self-learning and autonomous learning.

Integrated curriculum	A curriculum that mixes clinical and basic science teaching.
Learning approach	The intent with which the student approaches the learning process—either to understand or to memorize information.
Learning prerequisite	A piece of information or a skill that must be mastered before any further learning can take place.
Learning strategy	The studying technique adopted by students.
Learning style	The way in which students prefer to learn, reflecting differences in personalities and the way they process information.
Lecture	A teaching technique suitable for delivering information to a large group.
Logbook	A method of noting students' prior experience and competencies in the clinical setting (usually less bulky than a portfolio).
Marksheet	A form allowing examiners to award detailed marks to students on their performance.
MCQ	Multiple Choice Questions: an objective assessment technique for testing knowledge objectives.
Mentoring	One to one teaching which guides the learner in personal and professional development.
MEQ	Modified Essay Question: an assessment technique that allows the exploration of several facets of a developing clinical problem.
Motivation	The drive which makes students want to learn.
Norm referencing	The use of the performance of other students in the cohort to determine the pass mark (i.e. 20% will fail the exam).
Objective	A detailed statement of what a student will be able to do (derived from the syllabus).
Objective test	An assessment which reduces possibility of bias (either by dispensing with examiners, using checklists, or more than one examiner).
Oral examination (viva voce)	An assessment technique in which one or more examiners test students on their knowledge, understanding, communication skills, and ability to think under pressure.
OSCE	Objective Structured Clinical Examination: an assessment technique using multiple standardized items, to assess clinical and knowledge objectives.
Outcome	A statement of what a student will be expected to do at the end of the course (derived from the tasks a PRHO will need to do).
Pace	The speed at which a teaching session is delivered.
Passive learning	Exposure to a learning situation that does not involve the student.
PBL	Teaching technique using a clinical problem as the focus for student centred learning in the small group setting.

Pedagogy	The way in which children are taught.
Peer assessment	Assessment by fellow students (or teachers in evaluation activities).
Peer support	Personal and professional support of a teacher by colleagues.
Pitch	The level of difficulty of a teaching session.
PMP	Patient Management Problem: an assessment technique that allows the exploration of a developing clinical problem.
Portfolio	A collection of information about learning or experiences.
Prior knowledge	Information that the student possesses that forms a foundation on which new knowledge can be built.
Project	A short piece of individual or group research on a particular topic, presented in varied formats.
Protected time	Teaching while clinical responsibilities are covered by another clinician.
Rating scale	A technique allowing an assessor to make a quantitative judgment about how well an activity was achieved (either in an examination or an evaluation).
Reflection	Thinking about an experience with the intent of analysing its success or failure.
Reliability	A measure of the repeatability and objectivity of an assessment.
Role play	A teaching technique in which both students simulate a situation—commonly one will be the patient, while the other acts as a doctor.
Role modelling	Using the performance of the clinician as a guide for students' professional behaviours.
Schema	The units in which memory are ordered (associated with the work of Rumelhart).
Self-assessment	Personal assessment of the students own performance.
Self-directed learning	See independent learning.
Seminar	Flexibly used term for small group teaching (often of knowledge objectives).
Service setting	Teaching while continuing clinical work.
Session	A single teaching encounter.
Simulated patient (S.P.)	An actor who plays the part of the patient—usually to help students learn communication skills or in assessments.
Small group teaching	Teaching a group of around 3–12 students.
Spiral curriculum	A curriculum that continually revisits subjects at increasing levels of complexity (developed by Bruner).
Standard	A level at which students are expected to perform.
Stem	In an MCQ or EMQ, the initial statement of the problem.

Strategic learning	A learning approach that mixes deep and superficial approaches to maximize success in assessments.
Student centred learning	Learning in which students have control over the content and process of their teaching.
Student autonomy	Students taking control of content and process of their learning with responsibility for its outcome.
Summative assessment	Assessing learning with the aim of grading the students and feeding back information to the institution.
Surface learning	A learning approach in which students seek to memorize information.
Syllabus	A written statement of the content of the course. This may be framed in terms of objectives or outcomes.
Task analysis	A list of the actions that need to be completed to achieve a task.
Teacher centred learning	Learning in which the teacher determines the content and process of the teaching.
Teaching content	The knowledge, skills, or attitudes that you plan to teach.
Teaching plan	A method of summarizing the structure, timing, and content of a teaching session.
Teaching portfolio	A portfolio of teaching experience, usually including a reflective element showing evidence of teaching activity and professional development.
Teaching process	The way in which you teach a session.
Teaching style	The approach to teaching adopted by individual teachers.
Tutorial	Flexibly used term for small group teaching.
Validity	A measure of the degree to which an assessment covers the content of the course and measures what it is expected to test.

Index